Your Skin From
A to Z

Your Skin From *A to Z*

JEROME Z. LITT, M.D.

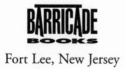
BARRICADE
BOOKS

Fort Lee, New Jersey

Published by Barricade Books Inc.
185 Bridge Plaza North
Suite 308-A
Ft. Lee, NJ 07024

Library of Congress Cataloging-in-Publication Data

Litt, Jerome Z.
    Your skin: from A to Z / Jerome Z. Litt.
        p. cm.
    ISBN: 1-56980-216-5
    1. Skin--Popular works. I. Title.

QP88.5 L55 2002
612.7'9--dc21   2001043042

First Printing
Printed in the United States of America

Contents

Introduction

THE SKIN

Not "skin." *The* skin. The house we live in.

When laid out flat, the skin of an average adult would measure some 20 square feet; it would weigh about 9 pounds. That's a lot of organ—one of the largest and heaviest of the body. It is also the most abused and maligned organ of the body.

Considering those "thousand natural shocks that [skin] is heir to," its continuing function and lack of complaint is nothing short of amazing.

How do we treat this remarkable mechanism? We dig and rub and scratch it. We expose it to all the elements—extremes of heat and cold, sun, wind, rain, and snow. We cut it, shave it, pick it, squeeze it, pinch it, and twist it. We scrub it, pull it, and bend it. We rub it, slap it, punch it, and knead it.

In the name of Beauty, we paint it and mark it and spray it. In the name of Health, we massage it and scorch it in the steam room and sauna. Name another organ that can stand up to all that! Yet it survives...

We never think of our skin as we do our heart, liver, lungs, kidneys, brain, or any other "important" organ. To many of us, this complex body stocking, worn so casually, is just a sac to hold our insides in, a bag containing some watery stuff and bones. And yet the skin is a vital, viable, living mechanism without which the human organism cannot survive.

- Think of what your skin, the most visible of all bodily organs and the only body tissue exposed to dry air, does to serve you:
- With its fifteen feet of blood vessels per square inch, your skin helps to regulate your body temperature, making it possible for you to adjust to extremes of cold and heat.
- Your large integument represents the first line of defense against harmful germs that constantly try to break through and invade your tissues.
- Despite its soft and elastic appearance, your skin is tough enough to withstand a variety of shocks and blows, acting as a cushion to protect delicate vital organs from harm.
- It is a porous yet leakproof organ, a protective barrier between your internal body systems and the hostile environment, preventing poisonous chemicals from penetrating your deeper tissues. At the same time, it prevents the outward loss of water, blood, minerals, hormones, and other essential body fluids. A genuine waterproof sac!
- Recent advances in dermatological research have shown that your skin helps to metabolize and detoxify certain drugs and potentially dangerous environmental chemicals. If a harmful substance lands on the skin and begins to penetrate, various enzymes will break it down into harmless constituents.
- Skin cells produce substances—interferons and interleukins—known to be important to the immune defense system.
- The skin is your largest organ of sensation, allowing you to perceive heat and cold, and various tactile impressions such as pain. It is the principal organ of communication between you and your environment—the "switchboard" that receives and transmits information such as "the stove is hot," "that knife is sharp," "this pillow is soft."
- It is an organ of excretion; a vast garbage disposal system continually eliminating body wastes through more than two million sweat pores.
- Your skin protects you against the harmful effects of the sun's rays by absorbing them and converting them into dark pigment (tan) to prevent further damage.
- Your skin is supplied with oil glands—100 per square inch—that

secrete sebum, the oily material responsible that maintains the resiliency and elasticity of the skin surface.

- The skin acts as a storage house for water as well as for various nutriments, such as sugar and calcium.
- It helps with the production of vitamin D (which is really a hormone). This controls the absorption of calcium and phosphorus—minerals vital for the development of strong bones, and for the prevention of rickets.
- Your skin is a mirror of what occurs beneath the surface—a warning signal of systemic diseases, such as diabetes, shingles, leukemia, and cancer, which often manifest themselves as skin problems long before there is positive evidence of the conditions internally.
- Your "decorative wrapping" is endowed with a special capacity to reflect human passions and sentiment. As a mirror of emotions the skin is without peer. Flushed with rage, pale with fright, blushing in shame, the sweating palm, an anxious pallor. All are release mechanisms of the skin that express a combination of inner feelings and skin reactions to tension, anxiety, and stress.

This, then, is your skin—"the envelope that encloses the letter of your biologic destiny"—that remarkable apparatus that spends a lifetime helping you adjust to your environment.

But we are not kind to our skin. We abuse it. And although we spend more than 20 billion dollars a year on skin care and cosmetics, we do not understand it. Only when the itching, burning or pain becomes unbearable, or when the cosmetic disfigurement becomes embarrassing do we begin to take it seriously.

Although the skin is strong and tough, it is also delicate and fragile. The cure-all in a jar that promises relief from such diverse conditions as acne, warts, eczema, dry skin, poison ivy dermatitis, genital herpes, and psoriasis is deceptive and misleading. One salve or lotion cannot be useful for a dozen different ailments, just as Cinderella's slipper will not fit every foot.

There are over two thousand different diseases and conditions that can affect the skin, hair, nails and mucous membranes. At one time or another, every person will develop some type of problem that deals with this large integumentary system. Warts, dandruff, dry skin, moles, athlete's foot. Excess hair or not enough hair. Rashes from the sun, from germs, from poison ivy. Insect bites, cold sores, hives, and rectal itch. Large pores, wrinkles, stretch marks or scars.

Famous figures throughout history suffered like anyone else:

- Job had boils.
- Caesar was bald. Queen Elizabeth I lost every hair on her body.
- Napoleon had scabies.
- Flannery O'Connor had lupus erythematosus and died of it.
- Tolstoy had canker sores. Wagner had eczema.
- John Updike has psoriasis. So did Ernest Hemingway.
- Winston Churchill had a persistent, intolerable, dry skin itch.
- Dr. Tom Dooley had a melanoma and died from it.
- Lyndon B. Johnson had skin cancer. So did Ronald and Nancy Reagan.
- Former Soviet leader, Mikhail S. Gorbachev has a large birthmark on his scalp.
- Golda Meir, Arthur Rubinstein and Richard Nixon suffered from severe shingles.
- Telly Savalas had a mole. Elizabeth Taylor and Madonna have moles.
- Michael Jackson has vitiligo.

Tens of millions of people all over the world have acne, warts, and eczema.

Your male friends may have hair loss, athlete's foot, or jock itch; your female friends may complain of large pores and stretch marks. And almost all adult women have cellulite!

Your children will have impetigo, diaper rash, ringworm, acne, warts, cradle cap, birthmarks, and insect bites.

Your parents will develop dry skin, wrinkles, skin tumors, leg ulcers, and shingles.

And how many of you are plagued with canker sores? Rectal itch? What about the more than eight million Americans who have psoriasis? And the countless millions frustrated by eczema?

No one can escape.

WHAT THIS BOOK CAN DO FOR YOU

In the following pages you'll learn about a few dozen conditions that commonly affect the skin, hair, and nails. Many of them are not diseases in the sense that they cause some bodily dysfunction, but are important enough to affect your general well-being and psychological health. You'll learn something about the causes and symptoms of these disorders, as well as different methods doctors use to treat them.

Please understand there is no magic in the treatment of skin disease. The skin, like every other organ, can develop "instant" maladies—ones that may take weeks or months to heal or improve. The sunburn that develops in an hour, the cold sores or poison ivy dermatitis that can begin overnight, the "zits" or boils that erupt in a day—all may take days or weeks of constant medication to get them under control.

A few of the products (or product-types) that I mention in these chapters are "over-the-counter" medications you can purchase at your local drugstore without a doctor's prescription. Some of these are "oral," medications that you take by mouth. Others are "topical" or "surface" medications that you apply directly on the area.

When using any medication, follow the directions on the label or the directions that I have provided. Be careful to note any special precautions. Different people respond differently to every medication, and its form, whether it's local, oral, or by injection. The salve that's so beneficial for Jason might cause Shelby to break out. The soothing lotion for Rachel might cause burning on Elizabeth's skin. And there are some people who, unfortunately, develop an allergy (sensitivity) to almost every variety of surface medications.

If you find that a preparation, whether over-the-counter or prescribed by a physician, causes an unpleasant symptom, such as burning, stinging, pain, or increased itching, discontinue it at once. It could be that you are—or have become—allergic to one or more of the ingredients in it. If this occurs, try a different type or brand of medication.

Lastly, do not hesitate to see your dermatologist. This book will not replace his or her expertise. Rather, it aims to help you better understand your skin and how to live in it.

For those who use the Internet, the following free websites will provide user-friendly links to a wide variety of skin problems and other medical topics:

www.lib.uiowa.edu/hardin
www.onhealth.com/
www.dermnet.org.nz/
www.mayohealth.org/
www.aad.org/
www.healthfinder.gov/
www.quackwatch.com/

Recap

- The skin is one of the largest and heaviest organs of the body.
- There are over two thousand different diseases and conditions that can affect the skin, hair, nails and mucous membranes.
- There is no magic in the treatment of skin disease. Like every other organ, it can develop "instant"" maladies—ones that may take weeks or months to heal or improve.

WHERE GOOD SKIN BEGINS

What does good skin look and feel like? Does the face or body of a fashion model or entertainment star pop into your head? Actually, glamour has nothing to do with it. You can't tell good skin by magazine photos or movie close-ups since photographers and makeup artists are trained to trick the eye.

Many psychological studies support the fact that people considered above average in attractiveness, and those who have clearer skin, earn more money. They attract better-looking and more successful mates, hold higher positions and find more opportunities than their less-attractive counterparts.

Your skin. Underneath it all, healthy skin is smooth, soft, elastic, fresh, and clear of blemishes. If that's not what you see when you look in a mirror, there may be a lot of reasons why not.

The way your skin looks and feels results from its condition and health. That depends on the following factors, some of which you can't control:

- Your heredity

- Your age
- Your general health
- Medications you may be taking
- Your diet (you are what you eat!)
- Exercise and rest
- How you take care of your skin
- Sun exposure
- Whether you're male or female

Heredity

Heredity plays a big part in what your skin is and what it will be. Black skin is thicker and tougher, has greater protection from the sun's dangerous rays, and wrinkles much less—and much later—than fair skin.

Black people, even when they're 70 or 80 years old, usually have fewer wrinkles than white people who are in their fifties. And, if a black person hasn't been in the sun a lot during his or her lifetime, you may *never* see a wrinkle.

If you are blue-eyed, blonde, and fair-skinned with Scandinavian or Irish relatives, your skin will usually be thin and delicate. This type of skin can't take exposure to the sun, wind, cold, or other harsh weather. It also develops wrinkles sooner than darker skin does.

Age

We're all getting older every day, but our skin ages differently depending on heredity, general health, and skin care. There are, however, some general stages in our skin's life.

Young people's skins are more delicate and thin than adults'. Infants have diaper rash and young children have scrapes, scratches, and bruises due to rough and tumble lifestyles, but also have less protection from the outside world than the adult whose skin has become toughened to the nicks and bumps of everyday living. The teenager whose oil-producing glands are increasing their activity will develop oily skin, oily hair, and acne.

When you get old, your skin becomes very thin and fragile, just as it was when you were a baby. Bumping your skin even a little bit can cause large bruises and blemishes. As your skin ages, it becomes saggy. Changes in hormones cut down the skin's oil supply and the skin becomes rough and dry. "Age spots" develop.

General Health

Your skin actually mirrors what's going on inside your body. So to have healthy skin, you must be in good physical and emotional health.

Many diseases, infections, and illnesses show up on the skin in several ways. For example, diabetes can cause dry skin, itching, pigment and nail changes, and yeast infections. Hepatitis and other liver disorders may create terrible itching or hives. Gall bladder trouble and some blood disorders will cause your skin to turn yellow. Hormone imbalances can change your skin color or make you lose your hair. Or cause you to grow too much hair. Certain blood diseases can cause itching, hives, and shingles, while lack of vitamins can bring on cracked lips, hair loss, dry skin, and mouth ulcers.

Stress, worry, and other emotional problems can show up as changes in your skin, such as acne pimples, hair loss, or differences in your skin's color, texture, or elasticity.

Medications

Taking vitamins, diet pills, and many other medications can change the appearance of your skin, hair, and nails. Very dry skin can result from taking thyroid medication and high doses of vitamin A.

Hives can develop from many medications. Usually aspirin, penicillin, and sulfa drugs such as those used for bladder infections (Bactrim and Septra to name only two) are responsible. Acne and oily skin are frequent side effects of low-dose birth control pills, anti-epilepsy medication (Dilantin and lithium are common offenders), and cortisone-like drugs. You can develop sun poisoning if you get too much sun while taking sulfa drugs, high-blood pressure pills, oral contraceptives, or medications of the tetracycline family. A rash that looks a lot like measles can show up if you're taking penicillin, ampicillin, sleeping pills, or scores of other medicines (See chapter on Drug Rashes). Low-dose birth control pills, thyroid medication, male hormones, high-blood pressure and lipid-lowering drugs, as well as most of the medications used to treat cancer, can cause hair to fall out.

All of these side effects shouldn't discourage you from taking your medicines, but you should know what *might* happen when you do. If you think you are developing an unusual reaction from some type of medication, check with the doctor who prescribed it.

Diet

Since the living cells that produce your skin, hair, and nails depend on what you eat for their supply of nutrients, it is important that you feed your body well. In other words, eat a well-balanced diet.

Poor eating habits can cause temporary hair loss, cracks in the corners of your mouth, and changes in your nails. Your skin may bruise easily, heal slowly, and look dull, drab, and "ashy." A good diet keeps your skin healthy, helps your skin have good tone, texture, and color, and protects your skin from disease. You shouldn't have to take vitamin supplements if you eat properly. There is no proof that swallowing extra vitamins or minerals does anything good for your skin.

Certain foods cause rashes and other problems. If you're allergic to penicillin, some cheeses (such as Roquefort and blue) can cause hives. If you like seaweed salad, you should know that kelp could cause zits. Eating too many carrots, oranges, or tomatoes can turn your skin yellow. Quinine (in quinine water) can cause bruising, blisters and hives. Seafood, chocolate, strawberries, and many other foods can bring on bouts of cold sores on the lips.

Exercise & Rest

Regular exercise is an important part of staying healthy. It cures boredom, tension, and anxiety, keeps your body in good shape, and enhances the color and texture of your skin. Exercising improves the circulation of the blood that then provides nourishment to the skin to build new cells, encourages the expulsion of impurities, and keeps the skin looking healthy and glowing.

When you don't get enough rest, circulation is diminished and the skin receives less oxygen and nourishment. As a result, your skin may look dull or sallow, and acne or dark circles can appear under your eyes. Suggestion: get your beauty sleep.

How You Take Care Of Your Skin

The number ONE rule for having good, clear skin is to clean it the right way. A clean skin is a healthy skin.

Proper cleansing removes the irritating, poisonous agents and germs that could hurt your skin or, by absorption through the skin, actually cause harm to other parts of your body. There are many ways to clean it, but the good, old-fashioned soap and water routine is really the best, most efficient, and least expensive method.

What are some of the things you want to wash away to keep your skin clean and healthy-looking?

First of all, you have substances produced by your own body:

- Dead, horny cells from the upper layers of the skin. If these are not regularly washed off, your complexion will be dull and lifeless.
- Sweat from the millions of sweat glands all over your body. A lot of this sweat is responsible for body odor.
- Sebum, the oily material that gives the skin its softness and elasticity. When this oily substance builds up, acne pimples result.
- Ear wax and old hair and nail cells, just sitting on your skin, up to no good.

Then there are the substances coming from the environment:

- Pollutants found in the air, such as smoke, soot, dust, pollens, and exhaust fumes from cars, busses, and trucks.
- Materials around your workplace, such as grease and grime from gas stations and fast food restaurants.
- Things found in your own home. These could be paints, glues, resins, clothing, bedding, carpeting, house sprays—even belly-button lint!
- All the bottles, jars, and sprays of "who-knows-what" you apply to your skin by design, such as cosmetics, suntan lotions, perfumes, and surface medications.
- "Friendly" germs that normally live on your skin.

Regular washing with soap and water rinses and flushes this garbage away, cleans the pores, reduces odor, and cuts down the risk of infection and disease. Your clean skin will look soft, glowing, and healthy. Its circulation will improve, encouraging the growth of healthy cells, and your skin will breathe better. All this comes from simply washing your face three times a day.

A word on cleansing creams used mostly to remove makeup. While your makeup seems to disappear, you're actually left with an irritating combination of cream, leftover makeup, and impurities that were on the skin to begin with. This leftover mess not only irritates your skin but also can clog the pores, leading to blackheads and whiteheads. If you try to remove it with tissues, you only further clog the pore openings.

Let's face it; only soap and water will really get your skin clean. Washing your face three times a day with a mild, gentle soap is the most important advice I can give. If you want to take off makeup with a cleansing cream, follow it up with soap and water to get rid of all that mess.

The kind of soap you use on your face is a matter of personal choice, but watch out for the ones that are irritating or can't be completely rinsed off. The so-called cold cream soaps, although they are fairly mild and gentle, always leave a film of cold cream, plugging up the oil glands that are already working hard to get rid of their normal oil supply. The deodorant and antibacterial soaps can be especially irritating to facial skin because they leave behind a residue of chemicals to destroy germs. If you have a body odor problem, use deodorant soaps below the neck only.

Do your face a favor and use a mild, gentle soap or cleanser that does its cleansing job well, rinses off easily, and leaves nothing behind. Try any of the following:

Aquanil Cleanser
Cetaphil Cleanser or Bar
Moisturel Cleanser
Neutrogena Bar

The Amount of Sun Exposure You've Had

To keep your skin healthy, you must learn to protect it. And the most harmful agent you must protect it from is the sun. Damaging sunrays can cause wrinkles and skin cancer as well. They're really hard on people with light hair, blue eyes, and fair skin.

A golden, bronzed body is beautiful! We think it's healthy and desirable. But a tan is nothing more than your body's marvelous defense against the dangerous effects of the sun's harmful rays, the ones that lead to early aging of the skin, wrinkles and, ultimately, skin cancer.

You absolutely cannot tan without damaging your skin. Sun damage is cumulative and irreversible. Your skin is like a sponge, and a bank: it soaks up all those rays and stores them. Forever.

The best protection from the sun is to avoid it completely. Second best is to apply a good sunscreen with a Sun Protection Factor of at least 15. (Please see chapter on Sun.)

Female or Male

Health, color, textures, and strength of skin depends on one's sex.

The next time you're at the shopping mall or in a crowd, take a look at white couples in their fifties or sixties. If the man and woman are about the same age, the woman probably looks about ten years older than the man. Her facial skin will appear drier and less elastic, and she'll have more wrinkles. Why? Several reasons:

- Because of the male hormone (androgen), a man's dermis (the lower layer of the skin) is thicker than that of a woman. As a result of this extra thickness, he is better protected from weather such as wind and cold air. He is less likely to have aging damage from the sun. Women's thinner skin also may be damaged more by outside influences such as cosmetics, facial exercises, and massages.
- Men's collagen fibers (the fibers in the dermis—the lower layer of the skin—that give the skin its strength and elasticity) are more tightly packed. That's why men don't have droopy skin around the throat or little vertical lines on the upper lip.
- The same hormones that make men's skin thicker, make it oilier than women's giving it a more elastic, resilient and flexible look and feel.

If you understand all of these conditions that affect the health of your skin—and what you can and can't do about them—you'll be on the right road to taking care of that marvelous organ we call skin. And you really should...it has to last you a lifetime.

Recap

- Heredity largely determines what your skin is and what it will be. If you are black, your skin is stronger than that of a white person.
- Your skin actually mirrors what's going on inside your body. So to have healthy skin, you must be in good physical and emotional health.
- The number ONE rule for having good, clear skin is to clean it the right way. A clean skin is a healthy skin.

1 The Dermatologic Dozen

Some skin disorders are much more common than others. Acne, for example, will occur in nine out of ten teenagers, making it the most common skin ailment seen by the dermatologist—the specialist in medicine who is trained in diseases of the skin.

This section deals with the twelve most common dermatological complaints—what I refer to as The Dermatological Dozen. These occur with sufficient frequency to comprise at least 90 percent of a dermatologist's office practice.

ACNE

> "There is no single disease which causes more psychic trauma, more maladjustment between parents and children, more general insecurity and feelings of inferiority and greater sums of psychic suffering than does acne."

Acne, the scourge of adolescence, is more than skin deep. There are few skin ailments that cause as much physical and psychological anguish as this complex chemical mystery that affects almost 20 million people in the U.S. The market for prescription and over-the-counter acne medications is well over $1.5 billion dollars a year. However, there are no quick, magical cures for it.

By far the most common teenage skin disorder, acne usually begins at puberty, when oil glands in the skin enlarge and increase

21

the production of skin oil (sebum). This occurs as a result of rising hormones during adolescence. Ranging from simple pimples to angry boils, the unsightly blemishes that fall under the general heading of acne, will plague 9 out of 10 pubescent youngsters; an age when physical attractiveness becomes so important. And no one wants to be Number One on the "zit parade"...

Acne appears most frequently in the mid-teens when hormone levels increase and kick the skin's oil gland into overdrive, but can show up as early as age nine or ten. It usually continues into the twenties. It may appear transiently in the newborn and is often seen in women in their mid-thirties. The incidence of acne in adult women is now more than 50 percent compared to 35 percent in 1979. (Neutrogena recently had an ad campaign with the slogan "Unfortunately, acne stands out even more on an adult." This is not very comforting to "thirty- and forty-something" women.)

The condition appears earlier in girls but is more frequent and more severe in boys. Overall, blacks and Asians tend to have fewer and less severe acne problems.

There is a great deal of controversy concerning the causes of acne, but most dermatologists agree that the basic problem is an overproduction of the skin oil by enlarged oil glands. This condition is characteristic of the internal chemical changes that occur at puberty when the skin is adjusting to a greatly increased output of hormones.

These hormonal factors play significant roles in the onset of acne, and since oil gland activity and sebum production are under the control of androgens (male-type hormones), the role of these hormones is crucial. In men, the testes are the primary source of androgens' hormones, whereas in women they are produced both by the ovaries and the adrenal glands. Acne seems to be the result of the oil gland's sensitivity to these androgens or their derivatives.

Acne can also be hereditary. The children of parents who had severe acne during their teenage years often develop severe acne too.

Acne occurs on areas of the body where oil glands are the largest, most numerous, and most active: the face, chest, and back. Simply stated, these enlarged and overactive oil glands become clogged with oil and sticky skin cells, thus forming blackheads and whiteheads. (When a skin pore is closed and oil can't escape, the swelling is called a whitehead; when the skin pore isn't closed but is simply plugged up with dead cells and oil, it's called a blackhead. The dark color of the blackhead is *not* due to dirt: it is a result of pigment cells—melanin—in the upper layers of the skin.) The glands continue to manufacture oil that is unable to escape.

Bacteria, which are always on the skin in "friendly" and harmless numbers, set up housekeeping and begin to thrive in these trapped secretions. They then become "unfriendly" and harmful, causing infected pimples. These may lead to cysts (little sacs filled with fluid or cheesy material), which then break down to form scars.

Many external factors can aggravate acne. Anything that prevents the oily secretions from flowing freely out of the oversized oil gland, such as infrequent washing, long hair (particularly bangs), hairspray, mousses, gels and greasy hair dressings, moisturizers, and other cosmetics containing lanolin can further plug up the already clogged oil gland opening to produce new lesions. Youngsters working at gas stations or fast food restaurants, who are constantly exposed to greases and oils, are especially prone to acne flare-ups.

Another type of acne—acne mechanica—is an aftermath of physical irritation to specific areas, either resulting in or aggravating prior acne. A common example of this process is the development of acne over the forehead, chin and back in teenage football players as a result of wearing football helmets, chin straps and shoulder pads. These sources of friction, combined with heavy perspiration, block the oil gland openings and often give rise to acne lesions over the affected pressure areas. The so-called "hippie acne" of a previous era, refers to the acne that occurs under headbands. A new trend—"cell phone acne"—is a result of keeping cell phones virtually glued to one ear, preventing the oil glands over the cheek from discharging its oily secretions.

Other factors that can aggravate acne include hormonal disorders as well as drugs such as cortisone, iodides, lithium, vitamin B12, and anti-epilepsy medications. Young men who are taking anabolic steroids for bodybuilding are prone to the severe cystic type of acne that doesn't respond to conventional anti-acne medications. Young women often experience acne eruptions just before their menstrual periods. The "low-dose" birth control pills also are responsible for

23

acne in women who never had the problem as adolescents. Many women note a worsening—even an onset—of acne two or three months after having discontinued their oral contraceptive. This phenomenon can last as long as two years. Excessive brushing with a hairbrush or hair dryer attachment may cause persistent localized acne over the temples and forehead.

Acne usually lasts for several years and abates in the early 20s. Poor self-image can result from years of poor skin, leading to feelings of inferiority, insecurity, and inadequacy that undermine self-confidence. Acne has been shown to be associated with impaired academic and social functioning; it also affects employment status. After acne has burned itself out, it may leave permanent scars on the psyche as well as on the skin. Both subside with time, but if the skin scars are severe, they may benefit from further treatment in the form of dermabrasion, chemical peels, punch grafting, laser treatments, or collagen injections. Some of the well-known actors who have facial scars from acne are Bill Murray and F. Murray Abraham.

While there is no easy cure for acne, you can control it to lessen its severity and to prevent the pitting and scarring that arise from neglect and self-medication.

The key to acne therapy is to control the overactivity of the oil glands, shrink them if possible, and destroy the bacteria that are responsible for the infection. And the earlier you treat your acne, the better.

Here are a few general principles that can help prevent or control acne:

- Wash your face thoroughly at least three times daily.
- Don't pick, pop or squeeze. This may aggravate the condition and lead to infection and scarring.
- Shampoo your hair frequently—daily if at all possible.
- Keep your hair off your face and don't use hairsprays, mousses, gels or greasy hairdressings.
- Avoid greasy cosmetics. Choose only the oil-free, water-based varieties, the ones that claim to be "non-comedogenic" or "non-acnegenic."
- Avoid harsh, abrasive cleansers or exfoliating scrubs that can

increase inflammation.

- Avoid creamy suntan lotions.
- Facials are not recommended because the creams and lotions that are utilized force more oil into the already-clogged pores.
- Avoid emotional stress. The chemicals released by your body during anxious and stressful situations stimulate the adrenal gland to produce more of the male-type hormone (more so in women!), which, in turn, stimulates the overproduction of skin oil.
- Watch your diet. The role that diet plays in causing acne is controversial and debatable. I recommend that you eliminate chocolate, seafood, nuts, and cheeses, and that you limit milk to three glasses a day. Adult women especially should avoid nuts and peanut butter at all times!
- If your physician has prescribed an antibiotic, such as tetracycline, erythromycin, doxycycline or minocycline for your acne, do not take multiple-vitamin supplements containing iron. Iron interferes with the absorption of tetracycline and other antibiotics.

Some of the latest topical (surface) measures include tretinoin (Retin-A), adapalene (Differin), tazarotene (Tazorac), and products containing antibiotics in different forms (lotions, solutions, gels and "pads"). Many of the older topical treatments that your physician might recommend include benzoyl peroxide (BPO), sulfur, resorcinol, salicylic acid and sulfacetamide. An old standby that works very nicely is an over-the-counter product called Acnomel.

For some of the larger bumps—cysts—that do not resolve with oral and surface means, your dermatologist may choose to inject a cortisone-like material directly into the cysts to help them disappear more promptly.

No therapy really "cures" acne. New lesions can occur despite good management. It can be controlled, however, to lessen its severity and prevent scarring. Don't be discouraged if your progress is slow. If you are diligent, conscientious, and faithful with your treatment, you will reap the benefit of a clearer complexion.

It is especially important that parents try to understand their teenagers' plight. By offering encouragement and helping your teenager maintain his or her self-esteem, you can help lessen the mental anguish and psychological scars that so often accompany acne.

Every day brings promise of a new magical cure. The best-heralded treatment for acne is an oral drug of the vitamin A family, isotretinoin. Sold under the name Accutane, this prescription medication works by shrinking the oil glands to reduce the output of skin oil. The Food and Drug Administration has approved Accutane for only the very severe and stubborn form of cystic acne that generally doesn't respond well to conventional forms of medication.

Accutane has many drawbacks. Pregnant women should not take Accutane because of the possibility of defects in the newborn. And women of childbearing age must show proof that they are not pregnant when they begin a course of Accutane treatments.

Accutane may also cause various undesirable side effects, including chapped lips, dry nose, dry mouth, dry skin, nosebleeds, and generalized itching. Other adverse reactions include muscular aches and pains, fatigue, headaches, conjunctivitis, blurred vision, and hair loss. These are temporary side effects, which disappear when the drug is discontinued.

Also, during Accutane therapy, blood tests must be taken every few weeks to determine the level of certain fatty substances—triglycerides—that often become elevated during therapy. Frequent follow-ups by your dermatologist are essential to monitor any side effects.

A relatively new oral contraceptive—birth control pill—Ortho Tri-Cyclen has been given the stamp of approval as being the only birth control pill that helps acne. Most all the others, the so-called "low-dose" pills, aggravate or actually trigger acne eruptions.

If your acne is stubborn, persistent, and disfiguring, consult your dermatologist. Waiting to "outgrow" acne can be a serious mistake; permanent scarring can result if acne is left untreated. A dermatologist can prescribe internal and topical medications to eliminate or lighten this cross that almost all teenagers have to bear.

For further information about acne, log on to www.aad.org
or phone: 1-888-462-DERM x22
Acne Support Groups:
www.m2w3.com/acne
www.familydoctor.org/healthfacts/001

ACNE—COMMON MYTHS & MISCONCEPTIONS

Myth #1: Acne is a disease of adolescence.

While it is true that acne usually appears during puberty, this is not always the case. Many people, particularly women, don't develop acne until their twenties or thirties, and it can afflict both men and women well into their forties.

Myth #2: Acne is more common in girls.

Young women are more likely to see a dermatologist about their acne problems because, as a rule, they are more conscious of their appearance. However, acne affects both sexes equally. As a matter of fact, the severe cystic form of acne of the back is more common in men.

Myth #3: Acne is due to improper hygiene.

In reality, acne patients generally are more fastidious and conscientious about cleanliness than other teenagers are. Blackheads, the primary hallmark of acne, do not result from dirt but from pigment (melanin) in the oil glands.

Myth #4: Masturbation causes or aggravates acne.

The only link between masturbation and acne is that both are often associated with adolescence. Moralists of the nineteenth century blamed many diseases on such "sinful" practices. The guilt surrounding masturbation in the minds of many teenagers probably perpetuates this timeworn myth.

Myth #5: Sexual intercourse will cure acne.

While this form of therapy sounds appealing, there is no evidence to document that it works. This belief probably stems from an old European myth that marriage cures acne. People often got married in their early 20s, about the same time that acne usually burns itself out.

A couple of notes on Zits: a zit is a colloquial expression that young people use to refer to acne bumps or pimples. Acne takes different shapes, named according to the size of the bumps.

Recap

- Don't pick, pop or squeeze your zits. This may aggravate the condition and lead to infection and scarring.
- Avoid emotional stress. The chemicals released by your body during anxious and stressful situations stimulate the adrenal gland to produce more of the male-type hormone (more so in women!), which, in turn, stimulates the overproduction of skin oil.
- Myth: Sexual intercourse will cure acne. While this form of therapy sounds appealing, there is no evidence to document that it works. This belief probably stems from an old European myth that marriage cures acne. People often got married in their early twenties, about the same time that acne usually burns itself out.

A couple of notes on Zits: a zit is a colloquial expression that young people use to refer to acne bumps or pimples. Acne takes different shapes, named according to the size of the bumps.

WARTS

We can travel to the moon, to Mars, to Venus, to Jupiter. We can annihilate polio, smallpox, syphilis, malaria, and scores of other disease entities. But we still cannot eradicate the common virus that's responsible for warts.

Over 25 million people in this country have warts. The common belief that handling frogs or toads causes them is, of course, only a myth. Frogs and toads have their own problems. Warts are growths on the skin caused by members of the human papillomavirus family. These viral growths should be destroyed because they are contagious, unsightly, and occasionally painful.

You can pass warts on to others by direct or indirect contact, in such places as locker rooms, public shower stalls, gymnasium mats, and swimming pools. Very often, members of the same household are afflicted with warts. They can also spread on the same person by picking, scratching, shaving, or biting ones nails.

Warts come in many shapes and sizes and can turn up on different parts of the body. The common wart is a raised, rough, grayish-looking, painless growth. It can vary in size from a pinhead to a fairly large mass. While they may occur on any portion of the skin surface and mucous membranes, common warts are usually found on the fingers, hands, and soles of the feet.

Flat warts are smooth, flesh-colored, and slightly elevated. These matchhead-sized growths usually appear on the face and backs of hands of children and young adults. Genital warts are found in the moist areas of the genital and anal regions. Warts on the sole are called plantar warts. (Not "planter's warts," as some people are fond of saying, as if there were something agricultural or occupational about them.) These warts are the most stubborn variety and frequently resist all known treatments.

That there are dozens of widely proclaimed methods to eliminate warts attests to the fact that there is no definite remedy. Ideally, the treatment should be quick, safe, and painless. It should not produce unsightly or lasting scars.

Some doctors recommend managing warts by letting them manage themselves. If left untreated, many warts will disappear by themselves in about two years. This seems to be their natural history. Warty people, however, may not want to wait for any spontaneous cure, so they seek medical advice.

The methods physicians use to treat warts are about as varied as warts themselves. The type of treatment your doctor uses will depend upon your age, the location of your warts, and the size and number of warts to be treated.

In electrosurgery, the wart is burned off with an electric needle under a local anesthetic. Warts also can be chemically destroyed using various types of acids, plasters, and other chemicals. Other warts can be frozen off with liquid nitrogen at minus 320° Fahrenheit. Still other warts succumb to surgical excision (cutting the wart out under local anesthesia).

Some dermatologists paint on a drug called cantharidin. After the application of this "blister beetle" remedy, swelling forms under the wart in a week to ten days. The dermatologist can then trim away the dead part of this blister roof, usually removing the remainder of the wart with it.

One of the latest modes of therapy for large or stubborn warts is the pulsed dye laser, which selectively destroys the nutrient-providing blood vessels that support infected cells carrying the wart virus to the lower layers of the skin. Another relatively new treatment calls for injections of an anti-cancer drug, called bleomycin, into each of the warts. These injections are, unfortunately, somewhat painful and expensive.

Genital and anal warts—reported to be one of the fastest growing sexually-transmitted diseases in the world—are usually transmitted by sexual contact. It is essential to treat the patient's sexual partner, in order to prevent recurrences. These venereal-type warts respond to podophyllin—a resinous substance that a physician paints on the warty growths at weekly intervals, as well as a relatively new cream—an Immune Response Modifier—called imiquimod (Aldara) that patients apply on their own. Women with genital warts have an increased risk of cancer of the cervix and, therefore, should be treated and closely followed.

Some doctors (and some grandmothers) charm warts away by suggestive methods. These "witching" methods have worked in many individuals, particularly young, impressionable children, and they leave no scars, no matter how deep or long-standing the warts may have been. Regardless of how bizarre or ludicrous a treatment may sound, if the patient has faith in the "charmer," the warts usually will disappear. However, I do not recommend stealing a piece of beef or a dishrag as old wives' tales do.

A great deal of research is currently trying to determine why certain people get warts and why they often disappear spontaneously. If you can't ward off warts, see your doctor.

Treating Warts

For small, flat warts of the face and the backs of the hands, ask your pharmacist for the following:

Castor Oil (one ounce)

Directions: Apply to warts twice daily using a cotton-tipped applicator (Q-Tip).

For the common type of warts on your fingers, palms, feet, and other areas, use any of the following:

Occlusal-HP, Compound W, Dr. Scholl's Wart Medicine or any number of over-the-counter varnishes or pads, all of which con-

tain varying amounts of salicylic acid.
Directions: Apply as directed on the package.

Some dermatologists have been reporting good success with the nightly application of Aldara (see above) for the treatment of common warts of the fingers and soles.

There are also some reports of Tagamet (cimetidine) pills getting rid of warts in children, but you should consult with either your dermatologist or pediatrician to find out whether this mode is appropriate for your youngster and what the dosage should be.

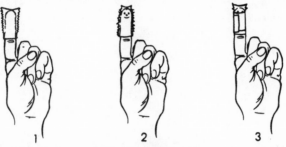

"Exorcising" Warts Using "Ducto-therapy"

For stubborn warts around and under the fingernails, use the following method that I call "ducto-therapy," using a roll of shiny duct tape cut in strips of one inch.

Completely wrap the wart with 2 "layers" of the duct tape. (See figure) Make it airtight. Do not wrap too tightly. Leave on for six days. Remove for half a day. Repeat the entire procedure—six days on, one day off. After several weeks, the wart becomes smaller, soft and mushy, gets "tired," and disappears, leaving no scar. Treat only one digit at a time; the largest first.

For more information on warts, log on to: www.aad.org
or phone: 1-888-462-DERM x22
or visit www.familydoctor.org/healthfacts/209.html

Some Folklore Remedies for Warts

- Take a dead black cat to a graveyard at midnight. When you hear a noise, throw the cat to ward the sound. That will take the warts away.

- Steal a greasy dishrag from your neighbor. Wipe your warts with it, and then throw it over your left shoulder into a pond.
- Rub warts with a raw potato, and then bury the potato in clay. Just to be on the safe side, repeat with another potato the following day.
- Rub warts with a black snail and impale the snail on a thorn tree. When the snail dries and withers, so do the warts.
- Rub the warts with a chicken gizzard during the waning of the moon. Then bury the gizzard in the center of a dirt road.
- Rub warts with a cinder, tie the cinder up in paper, and leave it at a crossroads. The finder catches the warts.
- Prick the wart with a gooseberry thorn that has been passed through a wedding ring.
- Lick your forefinger and point it at a passing funeral three times and say, "My warts go with you."
- Rub the wart with a piece of stolen beef. Bury the meat.

Recap

- Ideally, the treatment for warts should be quick, safe, and painless. And it should produce no unsightly or lasting scars.
- Women with genital warts have an increased risk of cancer of the cervix and should be closely monitored.
- Some doctors (and some grandmothers) charm warts away by suggestive methods. These "witching" methods have worked in many individuals, particularly young, impressionable children, and they leave no scars, no matter how deep or long-standing the warts may have been.

ECZEMA

"The patient with eczema is born to itch. He has the genes for itching as well as for asthma and hay fever."

Itch...scratch....
Itch...scratch...scratch....
In brief, this is the story of what people frequently call "eczema" and what dermatologists call "atopic dermatitis." It is a disease that

starts from scratch, and one that may last a lifetime. It is the eczema of infancy, the chronic, relentless dermatitis of childhood and adolescence, and the fierce and uncontrollable itching of the adult.

Eczema is a general term that, to most people, means a diffuse rash with itching. It is a synonym for dermatitis, literally "inflammation of the skin."

But when physicians speak of eczema, they usually refer to a persistent, incessant itchy eruption that almost invariably begins in infancy. It is inherited, and often accompanied in later years by hay fever or asthma. In rare circumstances it lasts a lifetime. It is atopic dermatitis, a disease that affects about 15 million people in the United States alone. The word *atopic* is used to describe eczema, asthma, allergic rhinitis, and hay fever. Often these diseases affect several members of the same family. The prevalence of eczema has nearly tripled since 1970 and it has been suggested that this increase is a result of environmental factors.

No one yet knows the "why" of this virtually uncontrollable, allergic process. It begins with itching on a perfectly normal-looking skin. You then rub, claw, tear, and scratch where it itches. You produce the rash we know of as eczema. Many sufferers have a reduced itch threshold; it seems to be a hallmark of the disorder.

There are three different types or "stages" of atopic dermatitis.

The infantile form This usually begins about six or eight weeks after birth. The itching is often intense and lasts up until about the age of two years. The rash, which almost always affects the cheeks and mouth, usually worsens after vaccinations and immunization injections, also during the teething phase. In the second year of life, the itchy areas develop over the hands, wrists, and outer portions of the arms and legs. Sixty percent of patients develop eczema in the first year of life.

The childhood type While the infantile form fades out in over half the cases between the ages of two and four, it may continue into the childhood type of eczema. The areas that suffer most are the creases in the elbows and the bends of the knees. Affected areas are drier, the skin thick and grayish, and the itching fierce. Children are restless, anxious, and hyperactive. Loss of sleep for young children suffering from eczema can diminish concentration at school and cause irritability.

Of all the eczemas that occur during childhood, atopic dermatitis is not only the most prevalent disorder but also one of the most mystifying and difficult to manage.

The adolescent and adult types The infantile and childhood eczemas often disappear after a few years only to reappear during late adolescence. While it usually fades away by the age of twenty, it may persist throughout the entire lifetime for some unfortunate people. The itching, again, may be intense and is usually worse at night. The areas affected are the bends of the elbows and knees, the face, the shoulders, and the upper back. The itchy and scratched skin becomes thick and leathery, darker than the surrounding skin, and develops dry scales. Many adult patients may have only chronic hand eczema.

Another characteristic feature is the accentuated groove beneath the lower eyelids. This is called the atopic pleat.

Triggering factors for certain people with atopic dermatitis include the following:

- Soaps and disinfectants
- Dust mites, pollens, molds, and animal dander
- Staphylococcal and yeast germs
- Foods, the most common of which are eggs, peanuts, milk, fish, citrus fruits, cheese and wheat
- Hormonal changes in women
- Sweating
- Perfumes and other scents
- "Nerves"
- Climate. In some patients, eczema worsens during the winter months. In others, during spring or fall.

The management of eczema is an enormous challenge for the physician. No one treatment works for everyone, since the areas involved and the degree of itching affect people in different ways. At best we try to alleviate the intense itching that, in essence, *is* the disease. Interrupting this fierce symptom breaks the itch-scratch reflex that is wholly responsible for the clinical manifestation—the rash.

Although there is no specific treatment for controlling eczema, here are some general measures:

- Never use soap! Soap removes the natural oils from your already dry skin. Use a soap free cleanser, such as Cetaphil.
- Take baths and showers in lukewarm—not hot—water. Add soothing bath oils to the water for excessively dry, scaly skin. And when you dry, do so by patting—not by rubbing.
- Keep fingernails short and clean.
- Avoid sudden extremes of temperature, and any violent exercise that causes sweating. Going from a hot to a cold or from a cold to a hot environment will trigger the itching mechanism.
- Keep the relative humidity above 40 percent—winter and summer—to protect the already dry skin from becoming completely dehydrated.
- Eliminate fuzzy, rough and woolen clothing, as these aggravate eczema. Soft, loose, cotton clothing is best.
- Get rid of furry toys and feather pillows.
- Do not allow children to play on floor rugs or rough upholstery.
- Unfortunately, removing household pets, particularly longhaired dogs and cats, is a must.
- Don't work around or expose yourself to dust, industrial chemicals, fumes, sprays, cutting oils, paints, varnishes, and solvents. All these will tend to worsen your eczema.
- Avoid all cosmetics, cleansers, body oils and lotions that contain lanolin. Lanolin is good for sheep but bad for humans. It causes allergies, plugs up oil glands (causing acne), and aggravates eczema. (Besides, why use a product on your skin that polishes shoes and cleans pots?)
- Try to avoid colds and other respiratory infections. These lower the resistance of your skin and make your atopic dermatitis worse.
- Don't wear rubber gloves for household chores. Even the cotton-lined varieties "sweat" when immersed in hot water, thereby leaching out chemicals and stabilizers in rubber that exacerbate eczema skin of the fingers and hands. If you must do the housework and dishes with rubber gloves, get cotton liners (Dermal Gloves) and wear them at all times under the cotton-lined rubber gloves.
- Avoid exposure to people who have cold sores (fever blisters). The virus that causes cold sores can cause serious eruptions in people who have eczema.

- Avoid over-the-counter salves and lotions containing benzocaine and antihistamines.
- Don't use Vaseline and other greasy ointments. These tend to intensify the itching by preventing the evaporation of sweat.
- During the winter holidays, steer clear of live Christmas trees. The artificial varieties are less irritating and less allergenic to eczema sufferers.
- If you're a long-standing sufferer and have the opportunity, move to a dry, warm place—like the Southwestern United States. High humidity often aggravates eczema.
- Diet is not a factor in most cases of eczema, but if you think your rash worsens with a certain food, eliminate it for a few weeks to see if your condition improves. Milk, cheese, wheat, citrus fruits, peanuts, fish, and eggs are potential irritants.
- Whenever possible, avoid emotional stress and tension. You may find that a flare-up of your condition was actually triggered by some conflict, anxiety, or stressful situation. There is no other skin condition where nerves play a greater role.
- Try not to scratch. Not only will scratching aggravate your condition, it can break and damage your skin, thus contributing to secondary bacterial infection.

For the milder cases of eczema, over-the-counter hydrocortisone creams along with an oral antihistamine (never use topical antihistamines and never use Neosporin!) might relieve some of the subjective manifestations of the disorder. But proper control belongs in the hands of a dermatologist.

Above all, try to be patient and keep a positive attitude. Despite the agony it can cause, eczema is not a serious disorder. If you can learn to live with it and keep the rash under control, chances are it will burn itself out of its own accord.

If, however, your rash persists and the itching is uncontrollable, see your dermatologist. He or she will be able to prescribe some time-tested remedies in the form of creams, lotions, cortisone-like drugs, ultraviolet light therapy in persistent cases and, perhaps, antibiotics if your rash becomes infected.

A new surface medication, by prescription only, is an

immunomodulator drug that has shown remarkable results in the treatment of atopic dermatitis. Called Protopic—the generic name of which is tacrolimus—it may prove a godsend for patients with longstanding eczema. Ask your dermatologist for the details of this innovative therapeutic "miracle."

Note: For itching, never use any surface medications containing neomycin or "-caine" derivatives, the most common being benzocaine.

For more information about eczema, contact:
National Eczema Association for Science & Education
1220 SW Morrison Suite 433, Portland, OR 97205
Tel: 1-800-818-7546 / 503-228-4430
or visit www.familydoctor.org/handouts/176.html
or www.aad.org
1-888-462-DERM x22

PSORIASIS

"Each morning, I vacuum my bed. My torture is skin deep: there is no pain, not even itching; we lepers live a long time, and are ironically healthy in other respects. Lusty, though we are loathsome to love. Keen-sighted, though we hate to look upon ourselves. The name of the disease, spiritually speaking, is Humiliation." John Updike. From the journal of a leper.
—*The New Yorker*
July 19, 1986, 28-33.

Psoriasis is a stubborn, chronic, and as yet incurable disease of the skin. Some eight million people—150,000 new cases annually—suffer from psoriasis in the United States alone. And they spend more than one billion dollars a year ($2,000 every minute!) to treat this ailment.

Psoriasis—the word comes from the Greek *psora*, which means itch—was considered a form of leprosy in biblical times. But this "disease of healthy people," doesn't threaten or shorten lives. It is neither an infection nor an allergy. It probably is not due to any vitamin or mineral deficiency. It doesn't leave scars or make you lose your hair. And, except in severe cases, it doesn't interfere with physical activities. (In fact, it may not even itch.) To the psoriasis sufferer, however, it can be a traumatic disorder leading to psychological difficulties, functional declines, disruption of lifestyle, and interpersonal problems. One study found that almost one quarter of psoriasis patients contemplated suicide because of their inability to cope with the disease.

Patches of raised, red skin covered by silvery-white scales characterize psoriasis. It can occur at any age, but commonly begins in young adulthood. Frequent flares and remissions mark psoriasis. It usually recurs at unpredictable intervals and may be worse in the winter. It is often precipitated or aggravated by physical or emotional stress, upper respiratory infections, strep throat, viral infections, AIDS, alcoholic beverages, obesity, certain oral medications (lithium, beta-blockers, ACE-inhibitors, and anti-malarial drugs are a few), and skin injuries such as scratches, cuts, and burns—including sunburn.

Psoriasis is not contagious. It does seem to run in families—about one-third of psoriatic patients have a family history of the condition—although the pattern of heredity is not clear. If both your parents have psoriasis, the chances are 50-50 that you, too, will inherit it. Psoriasis is also associated with a form of arthritis that affects the joints of the fingers. Up to thirty percent of people with psoriasis have symptoms of arthritis of various joints.

No one knows the cause of psoriasis, but we do know how it begins. Normal skin cells have a life span of about twenty-eight days. This is the time it takes for a cell to be born, move to the outer surface of the skin, and flake off.

In psoriasis the process goes awry due to some abnormality in the mechanism that makes the skin grow and replace itself. The skin cells develop, reproduce, and die at a rate ten times faster than the normal cells, causing a build-up of scales in thick, sharply-bordered patches. These layers of dead skin form silvery-looking plaques, which shed in clumps, leaving the skin underneath red and sore looking. These patches may be small or may cover the entire body. If they appear in the body's folds, they may cause itching and pain. Although psoriasis can affect any part of the skin, the patches usually occur on the elbows, knees, and scalp.

Psoriasis comes in many forms. For example, it can limit itself to the fingernails and toenails as small pits or stippling or loosening of the nails from their beds. In some unfortunate people, it affects the genital area and can limit sexual activity. In extreme cases, it is widespread, with painful cracks and total body redness and scaling, causing severe embarrassment. This, in turn, can lead to psychological problems; the true "heartbreak" of psoriasis.

Psoriasis is one of the most difficult chronic skin disorders to manage. Therapies that seem to be successful can suddenly cease being effective. Psoriasis can go into spontaneous remission and disappear, only to reappear abruptly.

If you have psoriasis, there are some remedies you can try yourself. But for serious or stubborn cases, I recommend you see your dermatologist. There are many treatments, old and new, which require a doctor's expertise.

The method of treatment depends on the extent and severity of the symptoms. An old standby is a tar preparation of the sort used with good results by thousands of psoriasis sufferers. Other methods are sunlight and ultraviolet radiation. There are also cortisone-like medications, which are applied or injected into the patches. These are the most widely used topical modality for psoriasis and generally work to reduce any associated itching.

There are various oral remedies that, while effective, may have potentially serious side effects. One of these is methotrexate, a drug that has been used for many years to treat difficult and extensive cases of psoriasis. Nausea, mouth ulcers, headaches, and harm to the liver or kidneys often complicate treatment with methotrexate.

Another powerful oral medication for severe psoriasis is a pill called acitretin (Soriatane). It is extremely effective for the severe, generalized forms of psoriasis, but there are many serious, adverse side effects. If you plan to enter into this therapy, make sure your dermatologist explains it to you. One of the latest treatments aims at regulating the immune system with cyclosporine (Neoral), a drug that's used as an immunosuppressant in organ transplant patients.

Every new treatment for psoriasis becomes headline news. Most of these "miracle treatments" quickly fall into disfavor or are discarded when another "breakthrough" surfaces. One of the earlier popular treatments—PUVA therapy—is aimed at slowing down excess cell reproduction. The patient swallows a relatively harmless drug called methoxsalen and then is exposed to longwave ultraviolet light. The proponents of this therapy swear by it, and today it has become a fairly common treatment for people with extensive psoriasis. There is some indication, however, that the PUVA treatment can lead to severe skin damage many years later. Another reported treatment, called climatotherapy, consists of bathing in the Dead Sea!

One of the recent developments in the topical treatment of psoriasis is a relative of vitamin D, which acts by slowing the growth of excessive skin cells and cell division. Called calcipotriene, this entirely new class of medication has gained fairly widespread acceptance for managing patches of psoriasis. In many published clinical trials, calcipotriene—trade name Dovonex Cream and Ointment—has compared favorably with many cortisone-like surface medications. Dozens of clinical studies have vouched for the safety and efficacy of calcipotriene in psoriasis. Another relatively new topical medication is tazoratene (Tazorac Gel) that also acts like the above-mentioned calcipotriene. Both Dovonex and Tazorac are prescription medications.

Another innovation is the "excimer laser," which purports "to produce a much more rapid response, making it much more convenient for the patient." But the jury is still out on this method.

For those of you who are discouraged by the progress of your treatments, be aware that more than forty experimental drugs are currently being tested to control this cosmetic scourge.

A stubborn form of psoriasis—on the scalp—occurs in about fifty percent of those suffering from the disorder. Difficulties in the treatment of scalp psoriasis arise because of the hair. Dermatologists usually recommend various shampoos, lotions and gels containing tar, salicylic acid, and cortisone-like products, but it's most important to shampoo on a daily basis. (This, needless to say, is often very difficult for women with scalp psoriasis.) A new topical mousse—Olux Foam—is another shampoo treatment with a novel delivery system that seems to cure the itching in a large percent of users.

But let's face it: while many of these treatments can help relieve the itching and scaling, there is no known "cure" for psoriasis. The cure will come about only when we know the exact nature and mechanism of the disease.

And while you must face the possibility that psoriasis will be a permanent guest in your life, let me offer some general guidelines to help you overcome the difficulties that accompany your condition:

- Avoid emotional stress and tension. Anxiety, anger, and depression commonly trigger psoriatic flares. Try to stay "cool."
- Keep clear of physical injuries to your skin, like scratches, cuts, and, especially, sunburn. If it itches, try not to scratch.
- When possible, prevent upper respiratory and other internal infections.
- When possible, eliminate medications that might aggravate psoriasis. Lithium, beta-blockers, certain ACE-inhibitors, Inderal, Indocin, and quinidine are common culprits.
- Try not to worry about what you consider the unsightly appearance of your rash. It looks a lot worse to you than it does to other people.
- Avoid those widely advertised "quick cures."
- Although diet plays a small role in psoriasis, I recommend that you limit your intake of red meat, poultry, eggs, dairy products, and alcoholic beverages for a few weeks to see if it helps. I know that doesn't leave much, but a temporary diet of fish and vegetables is a small price to pay for a chance at finding relief.
- Cooperate with your dermatologist.
- Don't be discouraged if progress is slow.
- And take comfort in knowing that with the variety of medications and treatments available, this potentially traumatic and hopeless disorder has a good chance of being controlled.

For further information about psoriasis, write to:
National Psoriasis Foundation
6600 SW 92nd Avenue—Suite 300
Portland, OR 97223-7915
800-723-9166; 503-244-7404
E-mail: getinfo@npfusa.org
www.psoriasis.org
www.aad.org/pamphlets/
1-888-462-DERM x22

Recap

- Psoriasis is also associated with a form of arthritis that affects the joints of the fingers. Up to thirty percent of people with psoriasis have symptoms of arthritis of various joints.
- Avoid emotional stress and tension. Anxiety, anger, and depression commonly trigger psoriatic flares. Try to stay "cool."
- Psoriasis is one of the most difficult of all chronic skin disorders to manage. Therapies that seem to be successful can suddenly stop being effective. Psoriasis can go into spontaneous remission and disappear, only to reappear just as abruptly.

DRY SKIN

June 8, 1955

"Found Winston in his bath in his most unreasonable mood."

"This tickle," he grunted, "is quite intolerable. It kept me awake. Yes, a bloody night. The skin man has given me fourteen ointments or lotions in turn without any theory behind any of them. Just doling out some potion or unguent to keep me quiet. It's a disgrace to the medical faculty."

"As the tenure of office of Winston's adviser seemed to be threatened, I had to explain to Winston that his skin had grown old with the rest of his tissues, and that none of us could put back the clock. He gave an impatient snort. He was not convinced. I explained to him that if he were willing to cut down the number of hot baths it might help the irritation of his skin very considerably. This he regarded as an outrageous suggestion."

—*Winston Churchill*
Taken from the *Diaries of Lord Moran*
(Boston: Houghton Mifflin, 1966)

Dry skin is a loose, unscientific term used to describe rough, scaly, and flaky skin—most often below the neck—that is less flexible or elastic than normal skin. And let me set the record straight: dry skin does *not* cause wrinkles.

Dryness of the skin usually develops as winter approaches. When the temperature drops and the relative humidity decreases, the upper layers of your skin lose a lot of water. This leads to dry skin with its scaling and occasional itching. This lowered humidity is further aggravated by artificial heating, which, in addition to warming the air, dries it. The dry, heated air expands like a sponge, sucking moisture from objects in the area, such as plants (withering), wood furniture (cracking, shrunken doors and creaky floors), and our skin. We usually notice the drop in relative humidity when we get those unexpected shocks from a buildup of static electricity.

Dry skin has a tendency to improve automatically during the summer months because perspiration keeps the skin moist as it reaches the skin's surface. When there is high relative humidity, there's less evaporation of moisture from our skin.

Dermatologists used to think that dry skin was caused by a lack of oily film on the surface of the skin. We now know that it's due to water loss from the skin's outer layers and the inability of moisture to move from the deeper layers to the surface. While the natural oils on the skin surface protect the water from evaporating out of the lower layers, these oils really can't prevent dry skin if there isn't enough moisture in the cells to begin with.

Several factors influence dry skin. It is more common in the elderly where, despite adequate water content of the skin, there are diminished oily secretions. Using harsh, alkaline soaps and soaking too long and too often in very hot baths can do it. Overheated homes with low humidity, as well as air-conditioning, which also lower relative humidity, likewise contribute to dry skin. Other factors include too much sunbathing, overexposure to wind and cold, fuzzy and woolen clothing, as well as nutritional problems and linens laundered in harsh detergents, improperly rinsed.

There are dozens of oral medications that can produce dry skin. Ask your physician or pharmacist, and look on the information sheets that come with almost all prescription drugs to find out if any of your medications might be among the culprits.

Here are some general guidelines for avoiding dry skin:

- Increase the relative humidity in your home to at least 40 percent by properly adjusting the heating or air-conditioning systems. If this is not practical, buy a good commercial room humidifier. Patients often ask me: "How do you know the relative humidity is 40 percent?" I tell them that when their windows fog up and wallpaper begins to peel, they cannot have dry skin! (I promise to replace the wallpaper.)
- Don't overheat your home. In the winter, keep room temperature as low as possible consistent with comfort. Cold winter air holds less moisture than warm air.
- Wash with a non-irritating cleanser such as Cetaphil.
- Use bath and shower additives. These will help keep the skin moisturized.
- When you bathe or shower, don't use extremely hot water or harsh soaps. Pat, do not rub your skin dry.
- Apply moisturizing creams or lotions—there are scores of them out there in the marketplace. Try one; try all. Find out which is the best one for you—on damp skin right after the shower or bath. This will help lock in the moisture in the upper layers of the skin.
- If you have hard water, consider installing a water-softening device.
- Avoid excessive sunbathing, cold temperatures, and strong winds.
- Don't wear heavy, woolen, fuzzy clothing.
- Do not sleep under electric blankets. This heat sucks out all the moisture from your skin.
- Keep healthy, make sure you eat a well-balanced diet, and drink plenty of water.

If you suffer from dry skin, try switching to mild gentle cleansers and use soothing bath oils and water-attracting creams and lotions that maintain your skin's natural moisture and leave it smooth, soft, and supple. The goal of dry skin therapy is to restore and maintain moisture in the skin, and the best way to treat dry skin is to prevent it in the first place.

For more information on dry skin, contact
www.aad.org
1-888-462-DERM x22

44

Recap

- Dry skin does not cause wrinkles.
- Increase the relative humidity in your home to at least 40 percent by properly adjusting the heating or air-conditioning systems. If this is not practicable, buy a good, commercial room humidifier.
- When you bathe or shower, don't use extremely hot water or harsh soaps. Pat, do not rub your skin dry.

COLD SORES & GENITAL HERPES

"She gallops night by night...
O'er ladies' lips, who straight on kisses dream, Which oft
the angry Mab with blisters plagues, Because their breaths
with sweetmeats tainted are."
—Shakespeare, *Romeo and Juliet,* 1.4.74

Like the common cold, cold sores are frequent, worldwide, and unresponsive to present-day treatments. They are also highly contagious, as the infection is spread primarily through social and sexual activities, usually involving close person-to-person contact. This, particularly in the case of genital herpes, can be most distressing.

Some people become infected from contact with eating and drinking utensils, from towels, and—yes—even from toilet seats! Close body contact in wrestling, rugby, and other sports can transmit the disease, and health care personnel are at special risk for infection of their fingers. Fortunately, cold sores are more irritating than they are dangerous.

The typical cold sore consists of a small group of water blisters on a red base. This blister group may itch, prickle, or burn. It can vary in size from that of a matchhead to a 25-cent piece or even larger. Although a cold sore can develop on any part of the body, it generally occurs on the mouth, the lips, or on the genital areas.

Up until a few years ago, doctors thought that cold sores of the mouth and lips—transmitted by contact with infected saliva—were invariably caused by a virus called herpesvirus Type 1. They also thought that cold sore-like infections below the waist—genital herpes—were always caused by a closely related organism, labeled herpesvirus Type 2. In recent years, due perhaps to a greater frequency in oral sex, the Type 1 viruses can cause genital "cold sores" and the Type 2 herpesvirus can cause mouth and lip lesions.

Cold Sores of the Mouth and Lips

Whether you call them cold sores, fever blisters, or the medical term herpes simplex, they all describe the same problem—a problem that can literally lead to a pain in the neck.

A virus causes cold sores. More than 40 million Americans suffer from them. The primary, or initial, infection with the herpes simplex virus usually occurs in early childhood. The infection, however, may not cause any symptoms for years while the virus lies dormant. Then suddenly, a variety of factors can trigger an outbreak of tiny clear, fluid-filled blisters—the visible sign of the infection. These factors include sun exposure, local injury (from dental work, for example), emotional tension, colds and other upper respiratory infections, various foods (chocolate, nuts, seafood), and, in rare instances, menstruation.

Ninety percent of the external lesions of cold sores will occur on the lips, while ten percent will develop on the nose, chin and cheeks. Often there may be tiny blisters over the gums or hard palate.

If left alone, the blisters rupture, the fluid inside begins to ooze and small ulcers develop. The ulcers then form crusts and scabs and finally heal in ten to fourteen days. As a rule, they do not leave scars but the virus that caused them remains in the body and migrates to nerve cells where it remains in a resting phase. If the infection is transmitted to the eyes, it can lead to blindness.

If there is excessive pain or discomfort and the lymph glands in the neck become swollen, it usually means that the virus has caused a secondary infection. When this happens, you may need an oral antibiotic.

Since cold sores are highly contagious, one should avoid kissing and sharing cups and lipsticks.

There's no cure for cold sores and fever blisters, but the recent introduction of oral and topical antiviral drugs for genital herpes (see below) and shingles, has prevented them. Many home remedies (a wet tea bag) and over-the-counter remedies are effective for cold sores of the mouth and lips.

Some common over-the-counter remedies that have been and are being used to ameliorate cold sores are Anbesol Gel, Blistex lip ointment, Campho-phenique, Herpecin-L, Viractin disappearing cream, and Zilactin medicated gel.

A relatively new, over-the-counter preparation called Abreva, has been approved of by the Food & Drug Administration to heal cold sores. Abreva—the generic name is docosanol—doesn't attack the virus directly. Apparently it alters the skin cells to create a barrier that prevents the virus from doing its harm.

A prescription ointment, penciclovir (Denavir), when used every two hours for four days, will usually alleviate the symptoms and help speed healing process for mouth and lip cold sores. For quicker and longer lasting "cures," oral anti-viral medications are the treatments of choice.

Consult your dermatologist if your cold sores are persistent or recurring. In extreme cases, herpes simplex can cause complications and lead to disease in the eyes, brain, and internal organs.

Genital Herpes

Genital herpes, or cold sores of the genital area, is considered a venereal disease because it is usually transmitted by sexual contact. Affecting more than 500,000 Americans each year, genital herpes is reportedly the most prevalent venereal disease among young Americans today, its incidence greater than both gonorrhea and syphilis. It accounts for about 15 percent of all sexually transmitted diseases in this country.

The threat of genital herpes has become so widespread that many young, unmarried Americans have altered their sexual behavior to prevent contracting the disease. And since the emotional, social and psychological impact of genital herpes is serious and long lasting, people are becoming more cautious about casual sex and thinking twice about the "one-night stand."

There has been a 30 percent increase in the prevalence of genital herpes since 1970; 22 percent of Americans over 12 years of age are infected, and is estimated to have affected more than 50 million people in the year 2000.

Like cold sores on the mouth and lips, a virus transmits genital herpes. This virus is usually transmitted by direct sexual contact (genital to genital or mouth to genital) with a person who has an active herpes infection. There is even the risk of contracting the herpes virus from a towel, drinking cup, or tester lipstick used by a person with open lesions. Given the opportunity, this virus can infect any portion of the body surface of a susceptible person. What is particularly disturbing are the unpredictable recurrences of these genital infections in the same person—at the same site—with a frequency that can be distressing, embarrassing and, at times, disabling. Fortunately, however, the herpes virus infections have a tendency to become milder with each recurrence.

How do you know if you have genital herpes? The average incubation period—that is, from the time of contact to when you first notice the symptoms—is roughly a week. Any number of signs and symptoms may precede or accompany a herpes infection of the genital region. These can include itching, mild burning and prickling sensations, pain during urination and sexual intercourse, fever, headache, and swollen lymph glands in the groin area.

Small groups of blisters commonly appear at the infected site—usually around the vagina or on the penis. These blisters break down in a few days, leaving shallow ulcers, which heal in about a week to ten days, when not complicated by infection.

For some people, a genital herpes infection is a painful, swollen inflammation. For others, the infection is relatively mild and transient, with few or no symptoms. People who are completely asymptomatic—and there are many—may act as reservoirs, or "carriers," for the disease, unknowingly affecting their sex partners. And so the question often posed by a spouse or a friend—"Who gave you (me) this herpes infection?"—cannot be answered with any certainty.

If you develop a herpes infection a week after sex relations, you have not necessarily contracted herpes from your sex partner. The friction of intercourse may very well have activated a dormant herpes virus in your body.

And while the primary infection (meaning the first time one is afflicted with the condition) is acquired by direct sexual contact (genital to genital or mouth to genital), recurrences of genital herpes infections are actually a reactivation of a latent, hidden virus, rather than reinfection.

What causes these reactivations—recurrences—and what are some of the triggering mechanisms? No one really knows.

After an active herpes episode, the virus remains quietly hidden in a nerve root, making treatment difficult or impossible. After weeks, months, or even years, the virus, stirred up by any number of mechanisms, travels down the nerve path and reappears on the skin, starting up a new batch of small blisters with all the symptoms of the earlier herpes infection. Some of the reactivating mechanisms that have been implicated in provoking recurrences include mechanical injury, masturbation, sexual intercourse, fever, gastrointestinal upsets, sunburn, fatigue, overexertion, sleeplessness, poor nutrition, menstruation, psychic stress, and even sauna baths!

Genital herpes is particularly disturbing because of its serious consequences. Extensive herpes of the genital organs can cause excruciating pain during urination and sexual intercourse.

The consequences for pregnant women are especially grim. Genital herpes is three times more common in pregnant women and results in a higher incidence of miscarriage and premature births.

Newborns who are infected during birth are unable to combat the virus with their immature immune systems. Thus, if an active genital herpes is present at the time of delivery, it can cause a devastating or fatal infection in the newborn as the infant passes through the birth canal. Therefore, most doctors recommend a Caesarean section for women who have an active herpes infection just before delivery.

In addition, women with genital herpes infections run a five times greater risk of cancer of the cervix. And for both women and men, there is a much higher incidence of other venereal infections, such as gonorrhea and syphilis.

There is a new test that takes just four hours to detect herpes simplex virus infections. This will help women avoid unnecessary Cesarean sections and it will help patients with herpes infections of the eye get prompt, often sight-saving, treatment.

While effective treatment for herpes is poor at best, you should

49

consult your physician to try to prevent complications that could lead to severe secondary bacterial infection and spread of the disease.

Treatment of the active infection consists mainly of relieving the symptoms:

- Reduce the inflammation and swelling with warm baths or continuous compresses using cool, whole milk.
- Relieve the pain and itching with aspirin, antihistamines, and appropriate topical medications prescribed by your physician.
- Control any secondary bacterial and yeast infection—again with medications prescribed by your doctor.
- Since urine can cause excruciating pain and stinging of vulvar lesions in women, protect that delicate area with zinc oxide paste.

As far as specific treatments for herpes, there are as many different kinds as there are doctors. Everything works...and nothing works.

Past and present treatments for cold sores have included applying cortisone-like antibiotic creams and ointments, ice cubes, ether, nail polish remover, liquid nitrogen, cortisone-type sprays, and a dozen different other topical (surface) medications. None of these treatments has yet withstood the test of time, but many doctors will still swear by their particular method.

One theory suggests that oral contraceptives help to prevent recurrences. There is also some evidence that the chemicals in most contraceptive foams have an antiviral effect on the genital herpes virus.

Proven treatments for genital herpes, include oral acyclovir (Zovirax), famciclovir (Famvir), and valacyclovir (Valtrex), all prescription medications. They all relieve the symptoms, reduce the shedding of the virus, and shorten the duration of an attack. They may also help to prevent recurrence of genital herpes. Valtrex has been shown to be far superior to topical measures for cold sores, since surface medications cannot penetrate the surface of the skin or mucous membranes where the virus is located.

Unfortunately, we cannot eradicate the virus by simply treating the local infection. For those of you who have genital herpes, I leave you with this sobering thought: you have it for life. And every time it recurs, it can potentially infect other people.

Here are a few suggestions, however, to prevent spread of the disease:

- Practice good genital hygiene; that means "soap and water."
- Wear soft, cotton clothing and avoid rubbing and chafing.
- If you are uncircumcised and prone to recurrent genital herpes, I recommend circumcision.
- When oral or genital lesions appear, don't have sex.
- Use a barrier method of contraception (condoms, spermicidal jellies, contraceptive foams, and diaphragm) if you are unsure whether you—or your partner—are actively infected.
- See your physician. He or she may suggest you take one of the oral anti-viral medications (as noted above) for months, years, or forever!

What does the future for herpes viral infections hold for us? If we will be able to produce a safe vaccine—such as those given to children in a single dose—then herpes, like polio, smallpox, influenza, typhoid, and diphtheria, will forever be eradicated.

We're working on it.

For further information about herpes, write to:
Herpes Resource Center
American Social Health Association (ASHA)
P.O. Box 13827—Research Triangle Park, NC 27709
800-230-6039; 919-361-8488
www.herpes.org or www.aad.org
1-888-462-DERM x22

Recap

- The primary, or initial, infection with the herpes simplex virus usually occurs in early childhood.
- Genital herpes is three times more common in pregnant women than in nonpregnant women and results in a higher incidence of miscarriage and premature births.
- When you have oral or genital lesions, don't have sex.

SHINGLES

> *"In Jerusalem, it was reported that Premier Golda Meir is over the worst of her shingles attack she suffered three weeks ago, but still has an irritating rash on her midriff. Doctors from as far away as California and Italy have offered diagnostic consultation to Mrs. Meir's physician and, according to the Jerusalem Post, sympathizers have been sending her medical advice and remedies for shingles through many Israeli embassies abroad."*
>
> —*New York Times,*
> January 24, 1975

Shingles (herpes zoster) is an inflammation of a nerve that causes pain, itching, rash, or all three. It affects an estimated 1.2 million people in the United States each year, usually in people aged fifty or older.

The word shingles comes from the Latin *cingulus* meaning a girdle. It has been known from biblical times as the creeping eruption that girdles the body.

Shingles has nothing to do with "nerves" in the emotional sense. You might hear someone say, "Oh! She's a nervous wreck. That's why she came down with the shingles." Nonsense. Because shingles affects a *nerve*, many people mistake this to mean that it is a nervous condition.

The condition has affected its share of celebrities—the late Golda Meir, Arthur Rubinstein, and President Nixon immediately come to mind—and such notoriety has led to misconceptions about it.

A virus causes shingles, the technical name for which is herpes zoster. It's the same virus that's responsible for chicken pox; it actually represents a reactivation of latent chicken pox viruses from an earlier infection. The virus remains in a quiescent state in certain nerve cells in the body and then reactivates, causing shingles. About twenty percent of those people who have had chicken pox will get shingles at some time in their lives.

No one knows why the virus "awakens" to cause shingles, but the prevailing theory is that there may be a temporary deficiency in the body's ability to fight off disease, such as may occur during periods of physical or emotional stress. This allows the shingles virus to pro-liferate and set up housekeeping along nerve fibers that reach toward the skin. Newborns, people taking cortisone-like drugs for long peri-ods, and those who have diseases that weaken the body's immune system, like AIDS, are highly susceptible to the shingles virus. Chemotherapeutic agents, radiation therapy, and drugs to prevent rejection of transplanted organs may also lower immunity to precip-itate shingles.

Like chicken pox, shingles is usually once-in-a-lifetime. Unlike chicken pox, however, it is only slightly contagious.

Although shingles can affect any age group, it's more prevalent and more painful in older people. And since shingles can attack any nerve, no area of the body surface is immune. Depending upon the severity of the pain and the location of the nerve involved, one can mistake shingles in its early stages for attacks of appendicitis, kidney stones, gallbladder trouble, pleurisy, and even facial neuralgia and toothache.

The virus of shingles attacks a nerve root in the brain or spinal cord and follows the course of that nerve only. Early symptoms include fatigue, headache, a slight fever, and a mild drawing pain over the involved area. The pain characteristically involves one side.

The infected areas of the skin become red and itchy, and a grouping of small blisters often follows along the path of the affect-ed nerve. These blisters last for about two weeks and then rupture, forming crusts and scabs that heal slowly.

Because each nerve extends to a very specific part of the body on either its left or right side, the blisters usually have a ribbon-like or branching configuration, forming a band in a semicircle on one side of the body.

In children and young adults, shingles usually runs a mild and quick course. In older people, however, the pain may be excruciat-ing, the itching may be intense, and the blisters may become crust-ed and infected.

Complications can arise from even the mildest form of shingles, so it is important that a physician examine any suspected case. Your doc-tor can prescribe various internal medications, such as antibiotics, cor-tisone-like drugs, analgesics and antihistamines, to relieve the pain, itching and inflammation, as well as soothing salves and ointments to relieve the dermatitis and possibly prevent spread of the disease.

When shingles involves the eye, you should consult an ophthalmologist (a physician who specializes in diseases of the eye) to prevent severe damage to the cornea. Arthur Rubinstein, one of the century's greatest pianists, had to retire from the concert stage in 1976, when an attack of shingles left him nearly blind.

Other complications of shingles that may occur are scarring where the blisters had been, extreme fatigue and malaise during the period of recovery. Also persistent dull or severe pain (postherpetic neuralgia) that may linger for months or after the rash has disappeared.

Occurring in more than half the patients over the age of 50, pain that follows an episode of herpes zoster can be extremely disabling. There have been a variety of attempts to control or reduce this relentless torment. They have met with variable success. A topical medication, capsaicin, may relieve some of this distressing symptom. This over-the-counter product, called Zostrix, should be applied 3 or 4 times a day, with relief of the pain anticipated in about 2 or 3 weeks. It should be continued for a period of several months, and for those who have been suffering from chronic pain, treatment over several years should be expected.

While there are no cures, as such, for shingles, many dermatologists have been prescribing any of three different antiviral medications to reduce the pain, to shorten the duration of the infection and, possibly, to diminish some of the complications. These oral medications are acyclovir (Zovirax), famciclovir (Famvir) and the newest "kid on the block," valacyclovir (Valtrex). Some dermatologists will often give a "cortisone" injection if the symptoms are relatively new. This, coupled with one of the oral medications, will frequently provide quick relief of the pain and itching.

It has also been shown that if valacyclovir (Valtrex) is given early enough—within a few days of the symptoms—the incidence of postherpetic neuralgia will be diminished.

One of the latest methods being used for relieving postherpetic pain is injecting the affected areas with European honeybee venom.

There are no measures known to prevent shingles. You may save yourself some worry, however, by avoiding direct contact with someone who has shingles. If you are older, and therefore more susceptible to shingles, you should also avoid young children who have chicken pox. Doctors will sometimes prescribe injections of gamma globulin for patients who are otherwise very ill and have been exposed to persons infected with either chicken pox or shingles.

If you do have shingles—some dermatologists call this "second-time" chicken pox—refrain from contact with infants and children who have never had chicken pox, and avoid people who are undergoing chemotherapy.

Shingles almost always limits itself to one side of the body. So, if you have a rash on both sides, chances are that shingles is not the culprit.

Some advice for those who have shingles:

- Over-the-counter pain relievers may help reduce some of the inflammation and pain.
- Wear light cotton clothing. Heavy fabrics that rub may increase pain.
- Warm baths are often helpful.
- Over-the-counter antihistamines can relieve much of the itching.
- For shingles on the face or scalp, and for any pain in the eye or ear, consult your dermatologist at once.

For more information about shingles, contact:
VZV Research Foundation
40 East 72nd Street, New York, NY 10021
www.glaxowellcome.com
www.healthylives.com or www.aad.org
1-888-462-DERM x22

Recap

- Shingles almost always limits itself to one side of the body. So, if you have a rash on both sides, chances are that shingles is not the culprit.
- Shingles has nothing to do with "nerves" in the emotional sense.

- Depending upon the severity of the pain and the location of the nerve involved, one can mistake shingles in its early stages for attacks of appendicitis, kidney stones, gall-bladder trouble, pleurisy, and even facial neuralgia and toothache.

INSECT BITES & STINGS

"The main of life is composed of small incidents and petty occurrences; of wishes for objects not remote; of insect vexations which sting us and fly away, impertinences which buzz a while about us, and are heard no more...."

—Samuel Johnson
The Rambler No.68

Spring and summer mean lush foliage, sunshine, flowers and... The Sting.

If you work or play in fields and gardens, bees, wasps, hornets, and yellow jackets buzz around loaded with nuisance, pain, and sometimes danger.

Bites and stings, for the most part, are only an annoyance and rarely cause more than slight, temporary discomfort. Either allergic mechanisms or sensitivity to certain chemicals, toxins, or enzymes in the venom causes the reactions to insect stings. Occasionally, these reactions can be fatal in sensitive individuals. Insect sting allergy has been recognized since antiquity. Hieroglyphics on the wall of the tomb of King Menes in Egypt record his death, in 2621 BCE, from a wasp or hornet sting. And today, there are more deaths in the United States from insect stings than from snakebites. Fortunately, mosquitoes cannot transmit HIV, the virus that causes AIDS.

The honeybee and yellow jacket are responsible for most stings. Although they may have similar appearances, these two insects have very different habits. The honeybee is a social insect that uses a stinger to inject venom into its victim. A yellow jacket is a wasp that can both bite and sting. The honeybee usually does not sting unless disturbed, but when sufficiently provoked to attack, it leaves its barbed stinger and attached venom sac in the skin of its victim.

It is often impossible to know when exposure to the responsible insect occurred, since skin reactions may not develop for up to nine days. The simple, normal sting, the one you are most likely to encounter, causes varying degrees of pain at the site of the sting, which last for a few minutes. Redness, swelling, and itching of the area follow. If no complications arise, all traces of the sting will usually disappear within a few hours.

In the exaggerated type of local reaction, there is more itching and swelling. The symptoms may last longer, and there may be a great deal of discomfort.

The treatment for most insect bites and stings is the same. In the case of a honeybee sting, however, you must remove the barbed stinger and attached venom sac as quickly as possible, as the walls of the sac contract and continue to inject venom. (Bumblebees, by the way, do not have barbed stingers, and thus may sting repeatedly.)

Never try to pull the stinger out or squeeze the area in which the stinger is embedded. This will break the venom sac, releasing more of the toxic or allergic substances and aggravating your symptoms. Instead, gently scrape the area with a knife blade or fingernail until the stinger and sac have been dislodged.

After you remove the stinger and venom sac, follow these steps to treat the simple insect sting:

- Wash the area with soap and water.
- Use ice packs or cold compresses for 30 to 45 minutes to reduce the inflammation.
- Apply a paste of one teaspoonful unseasoned meat tenderizer and water. This often provides prompt, lasting relief.
- Treat any hives and itching by applying Caladryl Lotion or Cort-Aid Cream every 3 or 4 hours.
- If severe swelling, itching, and pain persist, call your doctor. You may need an antihistamine or cortisone-like drug to counteract the bee venom.
- If you are stung on your foot or leg, elevate it and keep it at rest.

Insects are somewhat discriminating, so follow these steps to make yourself less of a target for bites and stings.

- Always wear shoes outside. Bare feet are the most vulnerable areas for insect attacks. Bees love clover and yellow jackets live in the ground.

- Avoid scented soaps, perfumes, colognes, hair sprays, and other scented products. These odors attract insects.
- Don't eat outdoors when bees are nearby.
- Since insects are attracted to carbon dioxide, do as little talking as possible at outdoor parties!
- Wear light colored, smooth fabrics. Bright, flowery prints and dark, rough clothing attracts insects as well. Avoid wearing blue.
- Avoid bright jewelry and other metal objects. Again, insects find these very alluring.
- If you come into contact with a stinging insect, avoid sudden and dramatic motions. Move away very slowly and do not flap, wave, or swat.
- Avoid touching insect nests. Honeybees usually attack people who disturb their colony.
- Keep house screens in good repair.
- Avoid stacking firewood and compost heaps against the house.
- Keep garbage cans covered at all times.
- Keep backyards clear of junk such as old tires and cans that can trap water and serve as a breeding ground for mosquitoes.
- Be especially alert after rain; pollen is scarce and insects become more easily excited.

A bit of trivia:

Only the female mosquito bites. Females need warm blood for the development and maturation of their young. Mosquitoes are twice as attractive to the color blue as to any other color and prefer warm body parts to cold ones. They avoid women who are menstruating. They can beat their wings up to 600 times a second, which is the source of the high-pitched hum we hear. And their activity increases more than 500 percent in the light of a full moon.

A word on insect repellents:

Insect repellents are not insecticides. They do not kill mosquitoes, ticks, chiggers, fleas, or the many varieties of biting flies. They just discourage them from biting you. And they do not work against stinging insects like bees, wasps, or ants.

To prevent against mosquito and fly bites, use insect repellents on exposed parts of your body and on your clothing. Do not use repellents on broken skin and be particularly careful when applying them on children. Pregnant women should not use them at any time. And since the active ingredient is flammable, do not apply them near fires.

For further information about insect bites, log on to:
www.aad.org
1-888-462-DERM x22

Recap

- There are more deaths in the United States from insect stings than from snakebites.
- In the case of a honeybee sting, never try to pull the stinger out or squeeze the area in which the stinger is embedded. This will break the venom sac, releasing more of the toxic or allergic substances and aggravating your symptoms.
- Always wear shoes outside. Bare feet are the most vulnerable areas for insect attacks. (Bees love clover and yellow jackets live in the ground.)

HIVES

"A disorder of hidden cause and unpredictable course."

Hives is a very common disorder. At least 20 percent of the general population will develop some form of hive-like eruption in the course of a lifetime. Fortunately, most episodes last for a few days to a couple of weeks and the cause, in these cases, is readily identified.

What are hives? Contrary to popular opinion, it is *not* a disease. Caused by the release of a chemical called histamine, hives—physicians call it urticaria—is a symptom of some disorder or allergic mechanism going on in the body. Hives appear on the skin and mucous membranes in the form of itching, stinging, and burning wheals (welts), surrounded by a zone of redness. They resemble big mosquito bites. New areas develop as old areas fade away. Hives come in a variety of sizes and shapes and can appear just about anywhere on your body, but mostly on pressure points: where you sit or lean.

When the wheals are very large and the loose tissue of the eyelids, lips and tongue swell up to form actual disfigurement, the condition is called angioedema, or "bull hives." Hives may involve the mucous membranes of the mouth and throat, and in rare cases may even obstruct breathing so severely that one requires heroic medical methods to prevent suffocation.

Like coughing or sneezing, which may signal a response to an upper respiratory infection or hay fever, hives are a clue, which alerts us to abnormal goings-on in our system. For example, it may be a response to an infection, an allergic reaction to some strange food or drug, or the result of emotional tension. It is extremely difficult to pinpoint the specific cause of a case of hives, because the possibilities are endless. It is somewhat easier to uncover the culprit in acute hives, the sort where the itching and wheals appear quickly and fade in a few minutes or hours. Among the possibilities are strange foods, an emotional upset, a penicillin injection, a new medication, and some recent infection such as chicken pox, mononucleosis, or an upper respiratory ailment.

Unfortunately, in the chronic form, the most common among middle-aged women, the cause is much more difficult to determine. It may last for months or even years.

The most common causes of hives are foods and drugs. Strawberries, nuts, chocolate, fish and shellfish, milk, eggs, pork, oranges, bananas, and other edibles, such as saccharin and aspartame, can cause hives. Hives can appear within minutes or up to two hours after ingesting the food.

Of the various drugs and medications, penicillin is probably the most common cause. If you are allergic to penicillin and suffer from hives, you should avoid milk and certain cheeses, such as blue cheese and Roquefort. Milk and other dairy products may contain enough penicillin to prolong hives for years. A woman who is allergic to penicillin may develop hives after having intercourse with a man who has been taking the drug. This phenomenon occurs because penicillin levels in semen can be as high as in the blood, causing the allergic reaction. The systematic use of other antibiotics, such as tetracycline, in cattle feed also can cause hives.

Sulfa drugs (sulfonamides) are notorious for causing hives. If you are allergic to sulfa (not sulfur), you should know that many common compounds contain sulfa. Saccharin and the "thiazide" diuretics—Lasix, hydrochlorothiazide, Prinizide and others—as well as the antibacterial drugs—Bactrim and Septra—can cause hives in those sensitive to sulfa. In addition, many vaginal creams, eyedrops (Ocusulf, Trusoft), acne medications (Sufacet-R, Novacet, Klaron Lotion, Plexion Cleanser), burn preparations such as Silvadine, cyclamates (Sucaryl, Sweeta, etc.), and most anti-diabetic drugs, such as Diabinese, Orinase and Glucotrol, contain sulfa!

Other classes of medication that cause hives are antibiotics, sedatives, tranquilizers, vitamins, laxatives, and dozens more.

Another common cause is aspirin. When you realize that Americans consume more than 25 million pounds of aspirin each year, it's little wonder that we see so many reactions to it.

Related to aspirin are other hive-producing chemicals known as salicylates. Salicylates appear in such products as root beer, wintergreen and mint flavorings, commercial bakery products, and mixes. Certain food dyes and preservatives (such as sodium benzoate), insulin, and various vaccines to protect against measles and polio may also be common offenders. So is menthol, found in such diverse products as cigarettes, toothpastes, candies, jellies, Noxzema, room deodorants, lozenges, and shaving creams.

Some people get hives from inhaling substances like animal dander (from cats, dogs, or horses), house dust, pollen, molds, certain plants, and flour in bakeries. Others break out in hives when they touch something cold or when they touch something hot and still others when they are exposed to sunlight. Some even get hives when pressure is applied to their skin, as in the shower.

There are certain types of hives that are of psychogenic origin. Fear, anger, and stress are the primary psychological factors responsible.

Underlying infections of the teeth, sinuses, gastrointestinal, respiratory, and genitourinary tracts all can cause hives. Hives is also associated with untreated athlete's foot and viral diseases such as hepatitis and infectious mononucleosis.

The treatment of hives consists of identifying and eliminating the cause of the condition. You—the patient—must be the detective.

What food did you eat? What medication did you take? Anything new? Anything different? Have you been to some strange place? What different inhalants or sprays have you been exposed to lately? Are you painting around the house? Have you mown the lawn? Are you experiencing emotional tension?

See your doctor if your hives are persistent, recurring, or severe. It is important that you provide as much information as possible to your physician. Only a physician can unearth the origin and nature of your hives, and only a physician can eradicate them. You may need a thorough physical examination, blood tests, X-rays, allergy testing, and other laboratory analyses to rule out any internal infection such as hepatitis.

For acute, temporary hives, over-the-counter oral antihistamines like Benadryl usually relieve the symptoms promptly—at least until your next exposure. If these don't work—or if they make you drowsy—prescription medications, such as Allegra, Claritin, or Zyrtec, might do the job. If the hives are severe and acute, see your doctor with all deliberate speed. He or she may have to give you an injection of adrenaline or a cortisone-like drug.

Finding the cause of chronic, recurrent hives is often a difficult, frustrating, and lengthy process, and requires patience and extensive detective work. Only when you are able to discover the cause, can you prevent your hives from recurring.

For more information on hives, log on to:
www.aad.org
1-888-462-DERM x22

Recap

- At least 20 percent of the general population will develop some form of hive-like eruption in the course of a lifetime.
- The most common causes of hives are certain foods and drugs.
- Of the various drugs and medications, penicillin is probably the most common cause of hives. If you are allergic to penicillin and suffer from hives, you should avoid milk and certain cheeses, especially blue cheese and Roquefort.

PITYRIASIS ROSEA

Pityriasis rosea is a most perplexing skin ailment. No one knows what causes it or what makes it disappear in a matter of weeks. We *do* know that it is usually a mild condition and that it is probably not contagious, even though small epidemics of the disease have occurred in Turkish baths, military establishments, and fraternity houses. If it is contagious, no one has been able to discover the germ that might be responsible.

Pityriasis rosea-like rashes can also occur in people taking various medications: penicillin, Accutane, Flagyl, barbiturates, beta-blockers, and others.

Commonly mistaken for ringworm, pityriasis rosea is a unique disorder. It usually begins as a single, large, round or oval pinkish patch, known as the "mother" or "herald" patch. The most common sites for this solitary lesion are the chest, the back, or the abdomen. This is followed in about two weeks by a blossoming of small, flat, oval, scaly patches of similar color usually distributed in a Christmas tree pattern over the chest and back.

This eruption seldom itches and usually limits itself to between the neck and knees. It is more common in adolescents and young adults and in the spring and autumn. It disappears as mysteriously as it came—the older lesions fading first—in about six to eight weeks, without leaving any marks or scars and without causing any complications. It rarely crops up in the same family at the same time, it is not a sign of ill health, and it doesn't affect the unborn children of pregnant women who are afflicted with it. And, it almost never recurs.

In other words, it's a pretty friendly skin condition!

There are, of course, exceptions, as there are in most skin diseases. For example, the herald plaque, which is supposed to signal the coming of a batch of smaller lesions, may be neither large nor conspicuous. Also, while the normal rash, at its peak, follows the Christmas tree pattern, it may cover the entire body. Occasionally, the condition brings on fierce and uncontrollable itching and, more rarely, fever, malaise, loss of appetite, and swollen lymph glands in the neck.

I have seen pityriasis rosea last for more than three months, and I have seen cases in the summer and winter. Several of my patients have been young children with intensely itchy "bumps" on not only the trunk but also the entire face and scalp, and I've even noted recurrences of this condition time and again. But, fortunately, these are only the exceptions. Usually, it is an extremely mild condition.

The treatment of pityriasis rosea is purely symptomatic: if it doesn't itch, leave it alone. If your itching is mild, soothing baths and an over-the-counter hydrocortisone cream or lotion applied two or three times daily should give you adequate relief. However, if the itching becomes intense and the rash begins to spread very rapidly, you should consult a dermatologist. He or she will prescribe appropriate oral medication and occasionally ultraviolet light treatments to relieve the itching and shorten the course of the disease.

One bit of advice: for your own peace of mind, don't take too much stock in nonprofessional opinions. Some people, seeing the sudden onset and spread of this strange rash, have shown it to relatives, friends, and the friendly pharmacist, who tell them that they probably have either ringworm, syphilis, AIDS, or some bizarre blood disorder. The most important consideration for those with pityriasis rosea is the reassurance that it isn't serious, contagious, infectious, or malignant. It will disappear in a matter of a few weeks without leaving permanent marks or scars.

For more information on pityriasis rosea, log on to:
www.aad.org
1-888-462-DERM x22

Recap

- Pityriasis rosea usually begins as a single, large, round or oval pinkish patch, known as the "mother" or "herald" patch. The most common sites for this solitary lesion are the chest, the back, or the abdomen.
- The treatment of pityriasis rosea is purely symptomatic: if it doesn't itch, leave it alone.
- Pityriasis rosea seldom itches and usually limits itself to areas

from the neck to the knees. It is more common in adolescents and young adults, and is prevalent during spring and autumn.

ALLERGY RASHES

More and more, people of all ages and from all walks of life are exposed to thousands of different substances that can affect the skin at home, work, or play. The enormous increase in the number of new chemical-containing products in the marketplace has been responsible for a large percentage of skin eruptions called contact dermatitis. It has been estimated that about eight percent of the entire population is affected at one time or another.

What do we mean by contact dermatitis? Simply stated, a contact dermatitis is a redness or inflammation of the skin that results from contact with a variety of natural or manufactured materials. The location and degree of inflammation depends on where the agent touched the skin.

The different types of contact dermatitis are divided into two categories: reaction due to irritation, or reaction due to allergy.

Recap

- An allergy develops when your body overreacts to a foreign substance. On the skin, it often takes the form of redness, itching, swelling, and sometimes blistering.
- A contact dermatitis is a redness or inflammation of the skin that results from actual contact with a variety of natural or manufactured materials.
- Just about one out of every ten patients who see a doctor for some skin problem will find out that he or she has an "allergic contact dermatitis."

Reactions Due To Irritation (Primary Irritants)

A primary irritant is a substance strong enough to cause a demonstrable reaction and physical damage to the skin in a high percentage of people, following initial exposure. The inflammation it causes may manifest itself merely as redness, or it may be severe enough to cause blistering and ulcers. It is similar in appearance to a mechanical injury or burn. Skin and deeper tissues are damaged, followed by inflammation and occasional scarring. How quickly the reaction occurs and how severe it is will depend upon the type of irritant, its concentration, the length of exposure time, and the degree of contact. Examples of strong primary irritants are lye, nitric acid, gasoline, turpentine, paint remover, and chemicals used for hair straightening.

These require only a few hours—or minutes, in some cases—to damage the skin. And they affect almost everybody. Mild irritants—soaps, solvents, laundry bleaches, and metal cleansers—affect a smaller percentage of people and may require several days of contact to produce an effect.

Irritations due to chemicals are treated like burns. The goal is to soothe, comfort, and prevent infection and scarring.

Reactions Due To Allergy (Hypersensitivity)

In simple medical terms, an allergy develops when your body overreacts to a foreign substance. Your immune system becomes hypersensitive to an allergen and then mounts an inflammatory tissue reaction to it. The reaction can take place in various parts of the body. In your respiratory system, it can show up as hay fever or asthma. In your intestinal tract, it may manifest itself as stomach cramps or pains. And in your nervous system, it can result in migraine headaches. On the skin, it often takes the form of redness, itching, swelling, and sometimes blistering. Why a person becomes sensitized to a material is not clear, but it appears to involve the person's immune system.

Just about one out of every ten patients who see a doctor for some skin problem will find out that he or she has an "allergic contact dermatitis." Unlike the primary irritant dermatitis, allergic contact dermatitis symptoms appear in a few days to a week. We can't predict who will and won't have an allergic reaction. Sometimes, a person could be touching the same material for many years without anything happening when suddenly he or she breaks out in a rash. Some people have allergies to a lot of different products they use everyday, while others use the very same products and never develop any signs of allergy. No one knows why.

There are myriad substances we come in contact with that could cause an allergic reaction no matter how healthy we are. To find the culprit requires good detective work. The majority of these substances are found in the home or marketplace. The following are some likely places to start the search:

Clothing:
- Wool, silk, furs, synthetic fibers, gloves, stockings, and underwear elastic.
- Clothing additives, such as formaldehyde resins, and finishes used to improve the look and feel of clothing—"wash and wear," permanent press, and antishrinkage/softening chemicals, especially the perfumed fabric softeners used in clothes dryers, such as Bounce and Cling-Free.
- Dyes—particularly the dark brown, dark blue, and black.
- Rubber materials, adhesives, chemicals used to tan leather, and shoe dyes. (A dermatitis on the top of the feet and toes is almost always due to an allergy to something in your footwear and not athlete's foot.)
- Leather goods, such as handbags, gloves, and wallets.
- Parts of clothing and jewelry containing nickel, including rings, necklaces, earrings, bra clasps, zippers, snaps, hairpins, and metal eyeglass frames.

Household Items:
- Glues, paints and varnishes, waxes and polishes, oil stains, plastics, soaps, detergents, and household cleansers.

Foods:
- Certain vegetables, fruit juices, and various spices.

Plants:
- Poison ivy, hyacinth, tulips, ragweed, etc.

Chemicals:
- Pesticides, insecticides, and fertilizers.

Over-the-counter drugs:
- Poison ivy remedies containing benzocaine and zirconium.

- Lotions and liniments to soothe burns, sunburn, and pain.
- Athlete's foot medications.
- Hair removal products for legs, underarms, and bikini areas.
- Analgesic balms and liniments for burns, sunburn, and pain.
- Depilatory agents.
- Tar preparations for psoriasis and eczema.
- Acne lotions, scrubs, and gels…and hundreds of others.

If you take a look at where a rash appears, you can usually figure out what might be the cause. For example, if the rash is on your face, you should suspect cosmetics—nose drops, sprays, eyeglass frames, and over-the-counter lotions, creams, and ointments. On the earlobes, consider earrings containing nickel (almost all do), hair dyes and sprays, perfumes, and other scented lotions. Necklaces, hair dyes and sprays, collars, scarves, etc. can cause a rash on the neck. In the armpits, consider antiperspirants and deodorants.

For contact dermatitis of your legs and feet, think of socks, stockings, pants, and shoes, as well as plants like poison ivy.

Colored or perfumed toilet paper, jock itch medication, feminine hygiene sprays, scented tampons, pads and panty liners, douches, hemorrhoid treatments, suppositories, and birth control creams and devices could cause irritation in the genital or anal area.

Some of the most stubborn allergies show up on the hands. Soaps, cleansers, detergents, gloves, plastics, and hundreds of metals, plants and chemicals could be the reason for the rash.

Some of the more common products responsible for allergic contact dermatitis are: nickel (found in almost all metal products including jewelry, particularly earrings), rubber (especially latex), chromium compounds (in cement, leather paints, shoes), and scores of others.

The following pages include a discussion of three common forms of contact dermatitis: poison ivy dermatitis, cosmetic contact dermatitis, and occupational dermatoses.

Poison Ivy Dermatitis

"Leaflets three, let it be."…is an old poetic warning. To which let me add my own unpoetic, "Don't be rash with poison ivy."

The three-leafer is the most common cause of contact dermatitis in the United States. More than 80 percent of all Americans are sensitive to plants of the poison ivy family. Poison ivy grows in most of the central and eastern parts of the country as low-lying shrubs or high-climbing aerial plants. It frequently appears under trees and poles and along fencerows. (It sometimes grows as ornamental shrubs in gardens!) The poison ivy plant has thin, pale stems upon which are three waxy, spade-shaped and pointed leaflets. (If you suspect that a plant is poison ivy, grasp it with a piece of folded white paper and crush it. If it's poison ivy, the sap on the paper will turn black in five minutes.) Poison ivy leaves turn red in the fall, and clusters of white berries form at their base.

Other related plants that can cause "poison" rashes are poison oak and poison sumac. Poison oak grows as a small shrub with clusters of yellow berries and the characteristic oak-like leaves; it is found mainly on the West Coast and accounts for 25 percent of all reported workmen's compensation cases among lumberjacks, utility line workers and firefighters. Poison sumac, flourishing in swamps and peat bogs along the eastern seaboard, grows as a tall, rangy shrub producing 7 to 13 leaves with cream-colored berries. The plants grow as vines on walls, fences, trees, telephone poles, and other vines, or as ground shrubs of various sizes.

Despite its name, poison ivy is not a poison. And, contrary to popular myth, the rash is not contagious. The sap of all these "poison" plants contains an allergic substance—one that can cause skin rashes in susceptible individuals. You get the rash by rubbing against or in some other manner exposing yourself to the plant. The allergic chemical in the plant—a sticky, colorless-to-yellow oil called *urushiol*—acts as a foreign material (antigen) on the skin, stirring up a defensive mechanism in your body. Your skin then forms "protective" cells (antibodies). This combination of the foreign and protective substances stimulates your immune system resulting in the redness, blisters, and itching that we call poison ivy dermatitis.

You don't have to come in direct contact with a poison ivy plant to develop a poison ivy rash. You can get it by touching shoes, various articles of clothing, sports equipment, and other objects that came in contact with poison ivy. You can get it by petting an animal whose fur may have been contaminated from bushes. The active ingredient in the poison ivy plant can remain active for months or years on inanimate objects, long enough to induce a rash if those substances are later touched. And you can get poison ivy dermatitis on your eyelids and face just by burning the leaves, due to active material in the smoke.

Following contact with the plant, a rash will develop in almost everyone. If you have a history of previous poison ivy episodes, then your rash can appear within a few hours after exposure. If you have never had poison ivy dermatitis before, the rash may take two to three weeks to develop after the initial exposure.

The rash that develops from poison ivy begins as redness, followed by small blisters, usually in streaks, accompanied by itching. The exposed areas of the skin—usually where the greatest amount of exposure has occurred—are most often affected: the hands, forearms, and face. The eruption may become severe, with marked swelling of the eyelids, widespread skin involvement, fever, and secondary infection.

Although poison ivy dermatitis is not contagious, the chemical responsible for the rash remains active after the initial contact. You can spread the rash to other parts of your body within the first hour after contact. After one hour on the skin, however, this chemical becomes neutral, and no further contamination will occur. Inanimate objects, such as clothing and camping equipment, can retain the substance for months, thus producing the rash when least expected.

Poison ivy dermatitis knows no season. More cases, however, occur in late spring and early summer, when the plant sap is most abundant in the stem and leaves. Your sensitivity to poison ivy changes with time and tends to decline with age.

Treatment for poison ivy dermatitis depends upon the severity of the eruption.

If you know you have come in contact with one of these "poison" plants, thoroughly wash yourself with a laundry detergent and water as soon after exposure as possible, preferably within ten minutes. While this will not prevent an outbreak of the rash, it may help minimize the spread. Make sure you wash under your fingernails, too. And wash all contaminated clothing, animals, and sports or garden equipment.

In mild, fairly localized cases, warm water compresses and plain calamine lotion (do not use other, over-the-counter "poison ivy remedies") will help dry up the tiny blisters and relieve the itching.

In more severe and extensive cases, it is advisable to see a dermatologist. The latest approved treatment, one that promises to stop the rash in its tracks, is high-dose therapy with cortisone-like drugs. This should be done early, as soon as the little bumps appear on the skin, and before the allergenic substance has a chance to sensitize the skin cells.

At the present time, there are no safe, approved methods of desensitizing people who are allergic to poison ivy.

The treatment for mild cases of poison ivy dermatitis is the same as the treatment for all allergy rashes. See page 000 for treatment.

To protect against these "poison" plants, first learn to recognize their physical characteristics so that you can avoid them when you are outdoors. In addition, wear protective clothing when hiking or weeding. Wear long sleeves, high socks, and gloves. *Never* burn poison ivy plants; the resin can be carried in the smoke and land on your skin or in your eyes.

Recap

- The three-leafer—poison ivy—is the most common cause of contact dermatitis in the United States. More than 80 percent of all Americans are sensitive to plants of the poison ivy family.
- Contrary to popular myth, poison ivy dermatitis is not contagious or infectious.

Allergy Rashes Due To Cosmetics

In our society we go to great lengths to look good and smell good. Myriad products on the market claiming to help us retain our youthful, healthy looks reinforce this pursuit.

The marketers of cosmetics prey on insecurity and legitimate health concerns, using various claims, which include the following:

"Hypoallergenic." All this means is that it doesn't have any fragrance, which is the most common cause of allergic rashes. Most cosmetics now proclaim that they are hypoallergenic.

- "Natural." First of all, why should "natural" products be better than laboratory-synthesized substances? They aren't! Then take a look at some of the so-called "natural" products and read the fine print on the label! In order for a product to stay on the shelf without becoming spoiled or rancid, preservatives must be utilized.

- "pH-Balanced." Almost all cosmetics and hair-care products are pH-Balanced, meaning that they are less alkaline and therefore less irritating than some deodorant bar soaps and strong alkaline shampoos.

- "Antiaging." All this means is that the product, usually a facial cosmetic, contains a sunscreen! Most of these antiaging cosmetics never list the sun protection factor (SPF), so you cannot know the relative degree of sun protection you are getting.

- "Rejuvenating." Another term for "wrinkle creams," this appellation is essentially meaningless. The ingredients for these "rejuvenating" creams vary, some including a sunscreen, others a moisturizer, and still others alpha-hydroxy acid components.

- "Environmental Protectant." Ostensibly formulated to protect the skin from the sun and pollutants, they may contain a sunscreen and various antioxidants such as vitamin C and E which, when topically applied, are essentially worthless, and provoke allergic dermatitis in many.

- "Dermatologist-tested." A meaningless claim, since all cosmetic products are ultimately checked by dermatologists who are either retained by the cosmetic company to help formulate the product, or solicited in trials to determine whether the product might be acceptable for some of their patients.

If you are a young woman, how many products might you put on your face, hair, body, and nails before you leave the house? From the top:

On your hair you might use conditioner, color or tint, shampoo, crème rinse, setting lotion, mousse, and hair spray. Dye? Bleach? Relaxer? Permanent-wave solution? In the bath you might use soap, bath oil, bath oil beads, bath salts, powder, and body lotion. And on your face—for starters—soap or cleansing cream and astringent, perhaps followed by moisturizer, foundation base, tinted base, shading cream, highlighting cream, contour cream, toner, freshener, clarifier, blusher, blotter, face powder, and mineral water spray.

Your eyes are next—eye shadow, eyeliner, eyebrow pencil, eyebrow powder, and mascara. Eye circle concealer? False eyelashes and glue? Lash extenders? For your lips—gloss, rouge, and lip liner. How about sunscreen? And how about a powder with "body glitter?" Aromatherapy products containing fragrance?

Your fingernails and toenails might require a cuticle cream, base coat, nail conditioner, nail hardener, nail lacquer, nail gloss, and/or quick-dry solution. Artificial nails, perhaps? And don't forget the depilatory, deodorant and antiperspirant, hand cream, feminine hygiene sprays, and perfume.

Cosmetic dermatitis is common in men, as well. The chief causes are shave creams, hair dyes, hair tonics, adhesives for hairpieces, bronzers, moisturizers, deodorants, soaps, sunscreens, and clear nail polish.

Then there are toothpastes, mouthwashes, whiteners, flavored floss....the list goes on and on.

Did I forget anything?

Would you believe that each product just mentioned—sixty-odd—could cause a skin allergy, hair breakage, or nail discoloration? There are about 8,000 chemicals that go into the making of cosmetics. You may use a cosmetic product for years without developing a reaction and suddenly become allergic to any of a number of the chemicals and preservatives, lanolin, dyes, and fragrances in it. In fact there isn't a product on the market, including the so-called hypoallergenic varieties, which cannot at some time, in some person, produce an allergic reaction on the skin.

A word about preservatives in cosmetics: Preservatives are necessary evils in all consumer merchandise. Without preservatives, cosmetics—and other products—would break down, spoil, and allow harmful germs to set up housekeeping. One of the common culprits in allergic rashes is formaldehyde, a disinfecting agent that many people have become allergic to. A very popular preservative in cosmetics is quaternium-15, a substance that releases formaldehyde thus triggering allergies. Other common allergens and irritants include: parabens, lanolin, acrylates and toluene sulfonamide/formaldehyde in nail cosmetics, paraphenylenediamine in permanent hair dyes, para-aminobenzoic acid (PABA) in sunscreens, and a host of others.

A rash—dermatitis—does not always occur over the area where you apply a cosmetic. Dermatitis of the eyelids or neck, for example, is often due to hand creams, nail polish or hair spray.

Cosmetic dermatitis is common in young men, as well. The chief causes are shave creams, hair dyes, hair tonics, adhesives for hairpieces, bronzers, moisturizers, deodorants, soaps, sunscreens, and clear nail polish.

How can you tell if you have an allergy to a cosmetic, and what can you do about it? Determine what new products you may have been exposed to just before your rash appeared, and then eliminate all possible irritants. Change soaps to a mild, white, perfume-free variety. (Cetaphil Cleanser or Bar are excellent soap substitutes.) Stop all scented lotions, creams, and sprays. Don't use any cosmetics for a week, and then gradually use them one at a time.

Or, better yet, try to live without a lot of them. The fewer the chemicals you expose your skin to, the less chance of it being irritated or sensitized. You should also consider external culprits. Have you been around anyone who wore a new perfume, cologne, or other scented toiletries? Anything new at the beauty shop or barber? At work? At school? The possibilities are infinite.

If you are unable to pinpoint the cause of your rash, your dermatologist will have the proper knowledge and equipment—patch testing, for example—to determine the cause. And unless you eliminate the cause, this allergy rash will forever plague you whenever you are exposed to your nemesis.

Recap

- There isn't a cosmetic product on the market, including those labeled hypoallergenic, that cannot produce an allergic reaction on the skin.

OCCUPATIONAL RASHES

At last count, there were almost 150 million people working in more than 70,000 forms of employment—a staggering number of occupations. And there are literally thousands of different chemical, physical and biological agents in these 70,000 occupations that can be responsible for contact dermatitis and other skin ailments.

The skin has many functions, not the least of which is to protect us from a hostile environment that includes germs, irritants, blows, chemicals, temperature changes, and radiation. Yet despite the ability of the skin to withstand many of these onslaughts, it is still the most commonly injured organ.

Here are a few facts:

- Almost never life-threatening, skin eruptions account for about 75 percent of all medical diseases compensated for and is the number one in-plant cause of lost time in industry.
- Fully ten percent of all skin diseases in the general population are work-related in origin.
- The cost of skin diseases due to occupational exposure runs into the hundreds of millions of dollars a year in medical expenses and lost time (on the average of 11 days a year per affected worker) on the job.
- Four out of 5 cases of occupational contact dermatitis involve only the hands.
- Those who have suffered from eczema in childhood tend to be more prone to occupational contact dermatitis than others. Their hands frequently become aggravated in occupations such as hairdressing and machine operating.

Occupational dermatitis is defined as a "contact dermatitis for which exposure at work can be shown to be the main cause or one of the factors contributing to its occurrence." Direct causes of occupational or industrial skin disease can be divided into seven groups:

1. Chemicals, the most frequent cause, include strong acids and alkalis, solvents, cutting oils, gases, and salts. All of these can injure the skin on direct contact, producing various kinds of rashes, while other chemicals, such as those found in leather, lacquer or rubber, can cause rashes that are allergic in nature.
2. Mechanical factors, caused by pressure or friction (prolonged use

of pneumatic tools, such as air hammers and chisels) are responsible for cuts, bruises, calluses, and the like. Fiberglas can produce a mechanical irritation and an itchy rash.

3. Physical agents in the form of excessive heat, sunlight, wind, and cold can cause burns, sunburn, allergic reactions, and frostbite.
4. Bacterial and fungal infections can occur among meat handlers, farmers, and grocers.
5. Insect bites and stings among outside workers are common dermatologic afflictions.
6. Bites from snakes and wild animals may arise in zookeepers, outdoor workers, garbage men, and mail handlers.
7. Poisonous plants and woods, as well as other vegetation, can cause skin problems among gardeners, farmers, road builders, surveyors, forestry workers, and telephone linemen.

There are hundreds of products and chemicals in industry that can cause dermatitis in otherwise healthy people. Almost anything can be responsible, but certain occupations are more susceptible than others to contact dermatitis.

The following are some common occupations and their materials:

Artists: Turpentine, solvents, clay, plaster, paint, sprays, ink.

Auto mechanics: Solvents, cutting oils, paints, cleansers, greases, kerosene, lacquer.

Bakers: Flour, spices, cinnamon, nuts, lemon, flavorings.

Barbers and hairdressers: Soaps, shampoos, permanent-wave solutions, hair dyes, rubber gloves, bleaching agents.

Bartenders: Detergents, cleansers, citrus fruits.

Bookbinders: Glue, plastics, solvents.

Building trades people: Cement, epoxy resins, rubber and leather gloves.

Butchers: Detergents, meats.

Canning industry: Juices, dyes, preservatives, brine.

Carpenters: Polishes, glue, solvents, cleansers, adhesives, wood.

Clerks and office workers: Carbon paper, glue, typewriter ribbons, copy paper, rubber, nickel, glutaraldehyde.

Cooks: Meat and vegetable juices, spices, detergents.

Dentists and dental technicians: Resins, acrylics, fluxes, mercury, rubber and latex gloves, local anesthetics.

Dry cleaners: Benzene, turpentine, carbon tetrachloride.

Electricians: Rubber, tape, glues, solvents, soldering flux.

Exterminators: Arsenic, DDT, formaldehyde, pyrethrum.

Florists and gardeners: Fertilizer, pesticides, plants (tulips, chrysanthemums, narcissus).

Food industry: Vegetables, spices, rubber gloves, detergents.

Foundry work: Oils, hand cleansers, resins, plastics.

Garment and millinery industries: Dyes, turpentine, benzene.

Groceries and delicatessen: Dyes on labels, insecticides, cardboard boxes, paper bags.

Hospital workers: Soaps, detergents, disinfectants, rubber gloves, penicillin, streptomycin.

Household workers: Detergents, polishes, solvents, rubber gloves, sprays.

Jewelers: Solvents, nickel, enamel, chrome.

Laundry workers: Detergents, bleaches, solvents, turpentine, starch, antiseptics, soap.

Manicurists: Nail polish, acrylic nails, cosmetics.

Masons: Cement, acids, resins, rubber and leather gloves.

Medical technicians and nurses: Detergents, plastics, solvents, antibiotics, antiseptics, anesthetics, formalin, rubber gloves.

Metal workers: Cutting oils, cleansers, solvents.

Painters: Turpentine, thinners, solvents, paints, dyes and adhesives in wallpaper.

Paper manufacturers: Glues and pastes.

Photographers: Acids, solvents, formaldehyde, dyes, color developers.

Plastic industry: Solvents, acids, additives, hardeners.

Platers: Solvents, paints, chromium, acids and alkalis.

Plumbers: Oils, hand cleansers, rubber, cement, nickel.

Printers: Solvents, glues, turpentine, paper finishes.

Rubber workers: Solvents, rubber, dyes, tars.

Shoemakers: Solvents, glues, leather, rubber, cement, polishes.

Sporting goods: Lead, rubber, nickel, chrome, leather, dyes.

Textile workers: Solvents, bleaching agents, fibers, dyes, finishes.

Theatrical profession: Cosmetics, dyes, glues.

Undertakers: Formaldehyde, embalming fluids.

Welders: Oil, chromium, nickel.

Window shade makers: Paint, benzene, shellac.
Woodworkers: Woods, turpentine, lacquers, varnish, tars, paints.

What is particularly sobering is that we can control and prevent fully *90 percent* of all occupational dermatoses by using protective clothing and cleansers.

The cure of contact dermatitis depends largely on detection and removal of the cause. This search for the causes can be one of the most intricate tasks confronting an allergist or dermatologist. But once we have discovered the causative agent, it is relatively easy to cure the rash and prevent recurrences.

For more information on various allergy rashes, log on to:
www.aad.org
1-888-462-DERM x22

Recap

- Skin eruptions account for about 75 percent of all medical diseases compensated for and are the number one in-plant cause of lost time in industry.
- The cost of skin diseases due to occupational exposure runs into the hundreds of millions of dollars a year in medical expenses and lost time on the job.

FUNGOUS INFECTIONS OF THE SKIN

Athlete's Foot

Athlete's foot does attack the feet, but it's not limited to athletes. It's also known as ringworm, but it's not a worm. Having dispelled two popular misconceptions about an ailment that affects so many of us, let's get down to the facts.

Athlete's foot is a nasty infection caused by a fungus. It occurs mostly among teenage and adult males. (You can call it a "guy" thing!) It is fairly easy to treat, but it can be stubborn, too. Although the majority of fungous infections of the skin are not life threatening, they can cause significant discomfort and embarrassment.

Fungous diseases, or disease caused by a fungus, are very common skin disorders. Fungi are living germs—actually miniature plants—that grow and multiply on the skin, in the hair, and in the nails of almost all living creatures.

(All fungi, by the way, are not harmful; many are beneficial and play a role in producing beer, cheese, and antibiotics such as penicillin. Other fungi, however, cause rust, mildew, and ringworm infections.)

Why some people develop fungous infections and others do not are questions that have yet to be resolved. Why females have a lower incidence is also unknown. Perhaps women are cleaner, sweat less, wash more often, and wear looser footgear. Maybe their hormones have antifungal properties. We really don't know. There is speculation that some people are immune to certain types of infections, and ringworm may be one of these.

Ringworm of the feet does not occur in primitive races accustomed to going barefoot, and it almost never appears in children under the age of twelve. Thus, if your child has a rash on his or her feet, it probably is *not* a fungous infection.

It is possible to be a host of the fungus of athlete's foot without any infection or other symptoms. It is only when you lower the natural resistance of the skin that the fungi thrive, proliferate, invade the outer layers of the skin, and set up housekeeping. This lowered resistance may be the result of excessive moisture and sweating (particularly in the summertime, due to sweaty socks and not drying your feet after swimming and bathing), inadequate ventilation of the feet (tight shoes and socks), uncleanliness, or friction. Athlete's foot is also very common in those who have diabetes.

Athlete's foot, the most common fungous infection affects people in different ways. For some peeling, cracking, and scaling of the skin between the toes, particularly the last two, characterizes it. Other people experience redness, scaling, and blisters along the sides and soles of the feet. Occasionally there is intense itching. It's also possible to develop a dry, reddish, non-itchy, scaly eruption, covering the entire sole. This common infection is referred to as the moccasin, or sandal, type of athlete's foot.

By the way, every rash on the foot is not necessarily athlete's foot. It may be an allergy from shoes or dye. It may be psoriasis, or any of a number of conditions that frequently attack the feet and toes.

If you have a persistent rash on your feet, consult your physician. Over-the-counter medications may only aggravate conditions that have been misdiagnosed as athlete's foot. If neglected, athlete's foot can lead to infection by other organisms—bacteria—that may require antibiotic therapy, continuous wet dressings, and complete bed rest. Only doctors can diagnose athlete's foot with any certainty.

How do you treat athlete's foot? No problem:

For simple, uncomplicated cases, I recommend applying antifungal creams or gels to the affected areas twice daily. This will usually cure the condition in a matter of weeks. If there is weeping, oozing, and blisters, and if the toewebs are wet and soggy, you should soak your feet twice a day in Burow's Solution before applying the antifungal medication.

If your athlete's foot is extensive, or has settled in your toenails, or if you have an allergic spread on your fingers and hands in the form of itchy water blisters, your doctor will probably prescribe some newer topical creams and lotions. Perhaps oral antifungal medications as well.

How can you prevent athlete's foot?

- Wash your feet at least once daily with soap and water.
- Keep your feet and toewebs meticulously dry at all times—use a blow dryer if necessary.
- If you are prone to athlete's foot, keep your toewebs separated at all times with one-inch-square pieces of cotton material (cut up an old shirt, sheet or handkerchief), but never use cotton batting. Or get some "toe-separators," sold in drug stores in the foot products section.
- Wear only 100 percent cotton socks and change them daily. Never wear socks that contain any synthetic materials; these are occlusive and cause sweating.
- Avoid tight or snug footwear in hot, humid weather (perforated shoes or sandals are best).
- Never go barefoot in a public shower or locker room.
- Always dry your feet well, particularly toewebs, with a clean towel.
- Dust an antifungal powder into your shoes in the summertime.
- Since your footwear can harbor these fungi (there is no effective

way to eradicate these organisms from footgear), it might be best to discard all your old shoes and buy a pair (or more) of new ones while treating your condition.

- Sandals are the best warm weather footwear.

Unfortunately, many people with athlete's foot suffer toenail involvement. About one third of all diabetics have toenail infection. If nail fungus is present in your toenails (and only your dermatologist or podiatrist can tell), you may have to treat these as well. If they are not taken care of, they act as a reservoir for subsequent foot infection.

If you follow all the suggestions mentioned above, athlete's foot will never trip you up.

Recap

- Ringworm of the feet does not occur in primitive races accustomed to going barefoot, and it almost never appears in children under the age of twelve.
- Every rash on the feet is not necessarily athlete's foot: it may be an allergy from shoes or dyes, it may be psoriasis, or any of a number of conditions that frequently attack the feet and toes.

"Ringworm"

"Ringworm"—actually ringworm of the skin other than in the scalp, beard, hands, feet, and groin—is a worldwide disease. The scientific terms for this prevalent disorder are *tinea corporis* and *tinea circinata*.

While it may affect people of all ages, it is most frequent in children. The source of the infection is usually a house pet (kitten or puppy), farm animal, or other infected child or adult.

The classic representation of "ringworm" is a sharply bordered, red patch ringed with tiny, blisters within which there appears a band of clearing. Central replication of this process, usually the rule in long-standing cases, results in the typical concentric rings that are considered the hallmarks of "ringworm."

As with other fungous infections of the skin—"athlete's foot," "jock itch," etc.—this form of ringworm is very itchy and occurs more often in hot, humid weather. Diabetes, obesity, and immune deficiency may predispose to more extensive lesions.

If you suspect that you or someone in your family has ringworm, see your physician with all deliberate speed. Since ringworm of the skin is highly communicable, treatment should be initiated at once. The application of an antifungal cream twice daily will often be sufficient to clear a mild infection in a matter of two or three weeks. When the lesions are more extensive and of long duration, your doctor will prescribe a course of oral antifungal medication.

If a household pet or other animals are suspected of transmitting the ailment, it would be prudent to have it checked by a veterinarian.

In all cases of ringworm, you should avoid sharing towels, linens, and clothing to prevent transmission of the infection.

Recap

- If a household pet or other animal is suspected of having transmitted ringworm, it would be prudent to have it checked by a veterinarian.
- In all cases of ringworm, you should avoid sharing towels, linens, and clothing to prevent transmission of the infection.

Ringworm of the Scalp

Ringworm of the scalp—tinea capitis—is the most common fungal infection in children.

Characterized by scaliness, crusting, itchiness and patchy hair loss, ringworm of the scalp is highly contagious, and sources of the infection are usually other children. In rare cases it can be caused by contact with a puppy or kitten. Hats, scarves, bandannas, headbands, pillowcases, and the like can spread this common infection.

Topical (surface) medication is not effective for this condition and your dermatologist or pediatrician will more than likely prescribe an oral medication to cure it. First a diagnosis should be made. This involves "planting" a suspicious hair from one of the patches onto a special type of medium—this is called a culture—and also looking at the suspected hair under a microscope to locate the culpable fungus organism. A prescription shampoo—Nizoral Shampoo (not the over-the-counter variety)—should also be used at least once daily.

Recap

- Ringworm of the scalp can be spread by hats, scarves, bandannas, headbands, pillowcases, and the like.

Jock Itch

Jock itch is one of those conditions, like hemorrhoids, that few people talk about in public. But there are a lot of people who suffer from it in private.

Jock itch is a common infection of the groin area in a young man that often occurs in association with athlete's foot. While the term "jock itch" is the popular expression that describes any rash in the groin area, it usually indicates a superficial fungous (ringworm) infection caused by the same organisms—miniature plants called fungi—that can give you athlete's foot.

Jock itch occurs more frequently in summertime. It commonly affects heavy people and those who are physically active. The tiny fungi that cause jock itch often live harmlessly on the skin, but when exposed to the right conditions—hot, humid, and damp places such as locker rooms, shower stalls, and swimming pools—they begin to thrive, multiply, and become harmful.

The groin area is more susceptible to skin irritation and infection than other parts of the body for several reasons. Groins are wet, warm, and dark. The skin is thin and delicate, and subject to friction, particularly if you do a lot of strenuous activity or if you have some extra folds of fat to chafe against your clothing.

Jockey shorts, tight pants, jock straps, and wet bathing suits not only make you sweat more, but prevent evaporation—making the groin area ideally suited for the growth and proliferation of these infectious organisms.

Jock itch usually begins as a small, reddish, scaly rash in the groin area that gradually enlarges to form a patch with a sharply defined border. If left untreated, the rash may spread to involve the upper inner thighs, the scrotum, the buttocks, and the pubic and anal areas. The skin becomes raw and soggy due to moisture and friction. Itching is the most common symptom, but there also may be some burning and pain.

How can you prevent jock itch? If you have it already, how can you treat it? Here are some general measures to prevent jock itch:

- Personal cleanliness (soap and water daily) is a must. Don't, however, scrub too hard. This may injure the upper layers of the skin and, as a result, compromise the body's natural defense mechanism that prevents invasion by harmful germs.
- After washing, rinse, and dry thoroughly. A blow dryer can help.
- Reduce perspiration.
- Help the sweat evaporate with proper ventilation. Wear loose fitting, cotton boxer shorts and loose pants. Air is a deterrent to the growth of these fungi.
- Change your underwear at least daily; it is a good breeding place for ringworm germs.
- Put your socks on *before* your undershorts. This will prevent dragging some of the fungi from your feet up to your groin.
- Wash your hands after touching your feet and toes.
- Don't wear anyone else's underwear.
- If you have a case of athlete's foot, treat it.

If you already have jock itch, over-the-counter ringworm preparations—also used for athlete's foot—can be applied twice daily. The chances are you also have athlete's foot, so treat this condition as well.

Recap

- If you have jock itch, put your socks on before your undershorts. This will prevent dragging some of the fungi from your feet up to your groin.

Candidiasis

Candidiasis—sometimes called moniliasis—is a common infection of the skin, mucous membranes, and nails (and, occasionally, internal organs) caused by a yeast-like fungus called Candida (or Monilia).

The body acts as a host to many different types of microorganisms including bacteria and fungi. Candida is a normal inhabitant of the human digestive tract where it flourishes without causing disease most of the time. While some microorganisms are useful to the body, others, as a result of a lowered resistance, can multiply rapidly, proliferate and set up housekeeping—very often on the skin.

These candidal organisms can involve almost any skin surface on the body and it is the most common cause of diaper rash in infants and young children where the warm, moist conditions under the diaper create an ideal environment for the proliferation of organisms. In adults it is often found in skin folds such as under the breasts, in the armpits, in the groin areas, in skin folds, around the nails, on the glans penis, and in the anal area. It is characterized by enlarging, scaly, reddish patches surrounding which are bright-red pimples and pus bumps.

Candidiasis often occurs during pregnancy, in diabetes, in obese individuals, in those who perspire freely, in those who are immunodeficient and due to various endocrine disorders. Other predisposing factors for candidiasis of the skin and mucous membranes include oral antibiotics and oral contraceptives, warm, humid climate, occlusion as with plastic and rubber panties (in babies) and nylon pantyhose, other underlying skin conditions, such as psoriasis, chemotherapy and corticosteroids, among others.

The condition called "thrush" is a form of oral candidiasis found in the mucous membranes of the mouth. It is very common in infants and young children.

Candidal infections are highly contagious and can be passed from direct contact, often sexual, or by contact from pets, clothing, showers, swimming pools, combs and the like.

Once your physician has made the diagnosis by microscopic or cultures examination (as is done for other fungal infections), topical, and occasionally systemic, treatment is simple and usually curative.

To prevent recurrences of candidiasis, keep the skin dry and preferably cool. Expose the affected areas to air whenever possible. Wear loose-fitting "breatheable" natural materials; wash hands thoroughly and often; and keep clothing scrupulously clean.

If you are taking an antibiotic, ask your physician to eliminate it for a few days, if it will not interfere with your general health.

And make sure you do not have diabetes. Only your physician can know that.

Recap

- To prevent recurrences of candidiasis, keep the skin dry and preferably cool. Expose the affected areas to air whenever possible. Wear loose-fitting "breathe-able" natural materials; wash hands thoroughly very often; and keep clothing scrupulously clean.

Tinea Versicolor

Tinea versicolor is a common, friendly, minor fungous, yeast-like infection of the upper layers of the skin. Friendly means that it is relatively harmless; minor means that it is only mildly contagious (through direct contact and clothing) and relatively easy to cure. It can be itchy and, when widespread, may be embarrassing cosmetically.

To the eye, tinea versicolor appears as fine, round, scaly patches that usually are tan or fawn-colored. These patches are most common over the chest and back or shoulders and upper arms. They can also appear on the neck, face and other areas of the body. Acting as a sunscreen, they block out the sun's rays. In white people, this results in depigmented areas of the skin. The patches are lighter than the surrounding tanned skin in summer and darker than the surrounding skin in winter. In black people, these depigmented patches can be various colors: tan, brown, gray, yellow, or even pink.

Like most fungous infections, tinea versicolor thrives in hot, humid environments. During the summer months, people often complain about itching and scaling; in winter, many of the symptoms disappear. Some people are more predisposed to this condition than others, and adolescents and young adults seem to be most susceptible. In tropical climes, where there is uninterrupted heat and humidity, people often have these patches all year round. In Liberia and Samoa, for example, almost half the adult population may be affected.

Tinea versicolor means "superficial fungous infection characterized by a change of color." To establish a diagnosis of this condition, a dermatologist will scrape some of the scales of one of the patches and search for the responsible fungus. Under the microscope, the fungus looks like a dish of spaghetti and meatballs—small spherical spores and rod-like filaments. (Dermatologists refer to it as the "spaghetti-and-meatball" fungus.)

The most common fungous infection in the world, *tinea versicolor* is easy to treat and leaves no scars. However, since the condition has a tendency to recur, particularly in humid weather, you may have to continue treatment over a long period of time. If left untreated, the condition may persist indefinitely.

Treatment usually consists of washing the affected areas with a non-prescription-type shampoo containing selenium sulfide (Selsun Blue) or ketoconazole (Nizoral), and applying a specific antifungal cream or lotion. Once you have begun treatment, it is important to wear freshly laundered or dry-cleaned clothing to prevent reinfection.

Many dermatologists are using some newer oral medications to treat tinea versicolor. Only a few tablets or capsules are required to destroy the infection, so if you have a stubborn and recurrent case of this "friendly fungus," see your dermatologist.

Even after you have destroyed the fungus, the patches may require repeated sun exposure—and Tincture of Time—to change back to their normal color. This may take months, so be patient!

For more information on the various fungous infections, log on to:
www.aad.org or www.familydoctor.org/handouts/316.html
1-888-462-DERM x22

Recap

- Although it's the most common fungous infection in the world, tinea versicolor is easy to treat and leaves no scars.

2 *Tumors of the Skin*

BENIGN TUMORS

A tumor is a swelling or new growth.

Tumors are mistakenly believed malignant by many people, but they include a wide variety of growths, both benign (friendly) and malignant (unfriendly), that can affect any organ of the body.

Benign tumors of the skin include warts, moles, skin tags, seborrheic keratoses, and molluscum growths. Common malignant skin tumors include the carcinomas (cancers) and the malignant melanoma.

Almost everyone will develop a skin tumor in his or her lifetime, but since the majority of skin tumors are benign and of little consequence, people rarely bring these to the attention of the physician.

Moles

"Under her breast
(Worthy the pressing) lies a mole right proud
Of that most delicate lodging."
—Shakespeare, *Cymbeline*, II, iv, 134

A mole, or "nevus," is a benign (friendly) tumor of the skin. Almost everybody has at least one mole—in fact, the average number of moles on the adult human body is about forty.

89

Moles are usually brown or brownish-black, but they may be skin-colored or pink or tan or even blue-black. They may be flat or raised, round or oval, single or in groups, smooth or warty, hairless or hairy. They can vary in size and shape, from a fraction of an inch in diameter to huge, irregular areas covering half the body.

We don't know what causes these tumors, but we do know that they run in families and that their presence is determined even before birth. In other words, if your parents have (or had) moles, chances are you will, too. What these moles will look like and where they'll occur, however, seems to be up to fate.

Most moles develop about the time of puberty or adolescence. They grow rapidly over a period of years and then slowly disappear—as if fading into the skin—in old age. Surprisingly, people in their seventies and eighties have very few moles.

The fashionable mole of a bygone era was fortuitous happenstance. Strategically located on a woman's cheek, people considered it a sign of beauty, and the name "beauty mark" is still heard today. Jean Harlow, Marilyn Monroe and Telly Savalas had moles. Elizabeth Taylor, Cindy Crawford, Arnold Schwarzenegger and Madonna have moles.

Other people, however, don't share this admiration for their own moles. The usual method for removing small moles is cutting them out under local anesthesia, a relatively simple and quick office procedure.

Although moles are harmless, they may change and become darker, causing concern. This can be due to exposure to the sun and to certain types of medications, such as cortisone. Hormone changes during puberty and pregnancy also may cause moles to become larger and darker and may even cause new ones to appear. More often than not, these changes are no cause for alarm. On rare occasions, however, changes in a mole can indicate a melanoma, the dreaded "black cancer." Although they are the most dangerous and fatal of skin cancers, melanomas have excellent cure rates if recognized early. They are removed by complete and wide excision.

So, if your mole suddenly becomes larger, changes in color or in texture, bleeds or crusts, or becomes itchy or painful, consult your dermatologist at once. Your doctor may recommend that the tumor be excised completely, or he or she may opt to surgically remove a small piece of tissue (known as a biopsy) and have it examined microscopically to determine the nature and extent of the apparent change. Most likely, your lesion will prove benign, but only a doctor can give you this reassurance.

For more information on moles, log on to: www.aad.org
or phone: 1-888-462-DERM x22

Recap

- Moles can vary in size and shape from a fraction of an inch to huge, irregular areas covering half the body.
- Most moles develop about the time of puberty or adolescence. They grow rapidly over a period of years and then slowly disappear—as if fading into the skin—in old age.
- If your mole suddenly becomes larger, changes in color or in texture, bleeds or crusts, or becomes itchy and painful, consult your dermatologist at once.

KERATOSES

Keratoses are tumors of the skin that occur in most people in the latter decades of life.

There are two kinds of keratoses, the most common being the harmless seborrheic keratoses. These are light brown, greasy, slightly raised growths that chiefly involve the face, chest, and back. They are slow growing, loosely attached to the skin, and are usually covered by a waxy-looking crust that appears to have a pasted-on appearance. They may be single or multiple and are usually round or oval, although they can take any shape. They vary in size from a fraction of an inch in diameter to up to half-dollar size or larger.

Some dermatologists call these "delayed birthmarks;" others, less kind, refer to them as the "barnacles of old age." I refer to them as the "barnacles of maturity."

Seborrheic keratoses appear to run in families. Unlike moles, they become more common and numerous with advancing age. They are not infectious or contagious, and never become malignant. Neither can they be prevented. Many people are fond of scraping these warty growths off with their fingernails—a habit I do not recommend. They may become infected, and invariably grow back if not completely destroyed. There are no curative or preventive internal remedies or salves/ointments that will rid a person of these warty growths. Some people choose to have them removed for cosmetic reasons.

Actinic keratoses, on the other hand, are very early skin cancers. And the offender in all cases is the sun. Also called solar keratoses, these tumors usually arise over the sun-exposed portions of the body—face, ears, forearms, neck, bald scalp, and backs of hands—and are commonly found in fair-haired, blue-eyed, fair-skinned people habitually exposed to the sun: the farmer, the sailor, the fisherman, the cattleman, the lifeguard. More than 100,000 new cases of actinic keratoses are diagnosed annually. Black people rarely develop actinic keratoses.

These tumors are rough, dry, reddish-brown, dirty looking growths firmly planted in the skin surface. If not treated, they may undergo serious malignant degeneration after many years. In other words, they become cancerous. When this happens, there is the danger of the disorder spreading to lymph glands and internal organs. Therefore, it is advisable to have these tumors removed before they degenerate into malignant lesions.

Your physician can remove both types of keratoses by any of the following methods:

- *Electrosurgery.* After the lesion has been anesthetized, the physician burns it with an electric current and then scrapes it off with a round knife called a dermal curette. Bleeding is insignificant, and the entire procedure takes but a few minutes. Depending upon the depth of the lesion, only minimal scarring results.
- *Curettage.* Following a local anesthetic, the lesion is scraped off in the same manner as described above, except there is no burning. Very small lesions may be destroyed by this method even without anesthesia, but this procedure is usually reserved for stoics.

- *Liquid nitrogen cryotherapy.* Considered the "gold standard" for the treatment of keratoses, this extremely cold substance (minus 320° F) is applied to the keratoses for a few seconds with a cotton applicator or a spray-type device. Over the next few days, the areas blister and the lesions become raised. They subsequently dry up and fall off. There is only minimal discomfort, and the cosmetic results are excellent. No scarring results from this method.

A physician can treat a dozen or more of these tumors by any of these methods, depending upon the size and location, without great inconvenience to the patient.

In addition, there is a chemical substance called 5-fluorouracil (5-FU) which, when locally applied for a period of a month or two, picks out the "disagreeable" cells of the more sinister actinic keratoses. This 5-FU—a self-administered topical treatment—produces a moderately severe reaction in the skin for a few weeks. After the process has reached its peak, the areas slowly heal, leaving the skin smooth and soft with no scarring. Dermatologists often recommend this procedure for multiple actinic keratoses, particularly about the face and scalp. (5-FU has no effect on seborrheic keratoses.) There are three brands of this topical 5-FU: Efudex, Fluoroplex, and Carac. All are prescription products.

A new system for the treatment of actinic keratoses is the Levulan Kerastick. This combines the application of a topical photosensitizer (aminolevulinic acid), in a "stick" form, with "blue light." Your dermatologist will be able to explain and discuss the various ramifications of this innovative therapy.

Other therapies involve full-face laser resurfacing; chemical peels; and the self-administered application of such diverse chemicals as alpha-hydroxy acids, Retin-A, Differin Gel and a whole host of other "cosmeceuticals" which have flooded the market. If you are confused, ask your dermatologist.

For those with a tendency to develop actinic keratoses—the fair-haired, blue-eyed, fair-skinned individuals—it is extremely important to avoid the sun. If your occupation, or hobby, requires sun exposure always use a sunscreen with a sun-protection factor (SPF) of at least 15.

For more information on keratoses, log on to: www.aad.org
or phone: 1-888-462-DERM x22

Recap

- Seborrheic keratoses become more common and more numerous with advancing age. They are not infectious or contagious, and they never become malignant.
- Actinic keratoses are very early skin cancers.
- For those with a tendency to develop actinic keratoses—the fair-haired, blue-eyed, fair-skinned individuals—it is extremely important to avoid the sun.

MALIGNANT TUMORS

Malignant tumors of the skin are the most common cancers of the human body. They are also the easiest forms of malignancy to treat. Almost 100 percent of all skin cancers—there are more than 1,000,000 new cases diagnosed each year—are completely curable.

Some of the well-known people who developed skin cancer are Ronald and Nancy Reagan, Richard Nixon, and Bill Clinton.

Since the skin is the largest and most exposed organ of the body, it is vulnerable to more environmental attacks from injury, weather, and sunlight than other organs. This coupled with exposure to various chemicals and industrial compounds, such as tar and arsenic, predispose our large "envelope" to malignant growths.

Because these tumors are directly visible and easily accessible, they offer a unique opportunity for early diagnosis, treatment, and cure.

The cause of skin cancer, like all cancers, remains a mystery but we do know a fair amount about the nature of the disease. Cancer of the skin occurs most frequently in fair-haired and fair-skinned people—those who lack adequate quantities of melanin, the pigment substance that filters out the deleterious rays of the sun. Most skin cancers develop on surfaces exposed to the sun. It is a common disease of farmers, sailors, fishermen, and athletes who spend a lifetime outdoors.

There are two common types of skin malignancies: the basal cell carcinoma and the squamous cell carcinoma.

The basal cell carcinoma, least aggressive of all cancers of the skin, grows very slowly and almost never spreads (metastasizes) to distant areas of the body. In its most common form, it is characterized by a pearly, waxy-looking nodule that may ulcerate after a period of time. It is what I call a "friendly" malignancy, and completely curable if destroyed before extensive growth has materialized. When left untreated, these slow-growing tumors invade and destroy the adjacent and deeper tissues, including bone. They rarely, if ever, occur in black people.

The squamous cell carcinoma, on the other hand, is a relatively dangerous tumor, one which, if allowed to grow, will involve the nearby lymph glands and internal organs. These cancers occur primarily on the sun-exposed areas of the face, rim of the ears, neck, and hands, and fortunately are much more rare than the basal cell type. It is rarely found in dark-skinned persons.

Early recognition and prompt, adequate treatment for all malignancies of the skin is essential. Early signs include any new growth that does not heal, or any *change* in an existing growth. If you have either of these signs see your physician at once.

If your dermatologist suspects "unfriendly" cells, she or he will surgically remove—under local anesthesia—a small piece of diseased tissue and have it examined microscopically for any possibility of malignancy. This procedure is known as a biopsy.

If the tumor is malignant, treatment will depend upon the location and size of the growth, the nature of the cancerous cells, and whether any spread is apparent. For the small, simple, "friendly" basal cell cancers, cauterization with an electric needle or surgical excision is a simple, quick, and safe procedure that can be performed in the doctor's office. Other methods include freezing techniques; locally applied chemicals that selectively eradicate the malignant cells; and the new laser treatments. Imiqimod (Aldara) is one of the latest surface medications being used for the treatment of small, non-facial basal cell cancers. Regardless of the type of therapy, healing is a slow process and scarring is an inevitable consequence.

In all cases and by whatever means, the physician must destroy or remove the entire tumor. Periodic follow-up by your physician is necessary to insure against recurrence of the lesion.

To prevent skin cancers, fair-skinned and sun-sensitive people should avoid unnecessary or excessive sun exposure. *Everyone* should use commercial sunscreens, with a sun-protection factor (SPF) of at least 15, to filter out the harmful and cancer-producing rays of the sun.

It's never too early—or too late—to stop this "quiet epidemic of the twenty-first century."

For more information on skin cancer, log on to www.aad.org
or phone 1-888-462-DERM x22
also contact:
The Skin Cancer Foundation
245 Fifth Avenue, Suite 1403, New York, NY 10016
800-754-6490; 212-725-5176
e-mail: info@skincancer.org

Recap

- Malignant tumors of the skin are the most common cancers of the human body. They are also the easiest forms of malignancy to treat.
- The basal cell cancer is a "friendly" malignancy and completely curable if destroyed before extensive growth has materialized.
- Early recognition and prompt treatment for all malignancies of the skin are essential. Early signs include any new growth that does not heal or any change in an existing growth.

MELANOMA

Evidence from many sources suggests a steadily rising incidence of malignant melanoma in the past few decades, accompanied by a rising death rate. Sam Donaldson and Troy Aikman have also been afflicted with these deadly tumors. Public figures suffering melanoma have increased public awareness of this deadly skin tumor. The mortality rate in the United States from the lethal growth is now over 9,000 a year, accounting for most of the deaths from skin cancer.

It is a malignant growth, which seems to appear out of nowhere, that invades adjoining tissue and distant organs, spreading via the blood and lymph channels.

Malignant melanomas are usually black lesions of the skin that arise in a pre-existing, dark, hairless mole—hence the epithet "black cancer." While occurring primarily on the skin surface, melanomas can also be pale and non-pigmented, and can appear in the eye, on mucous membranes, anywhere. No portion of the body and none of the organs are immune from this deadly tumor.

Unlike the other cancers of the skin—the basal cell and squamous cell carcinomas—melanoma has a striking tendency to spread to other parts of the body. Once melanoma cells extend to vital organs, they are much more difficult to treat.

While it can develop at any age, melanoma is seen most commonly in people between forty and seventy. The current ballpark figure predicts that approximately 50,000 men and women in the United States will be stricken this year. But this figure is greatly underestimated. As a result of gross underreporting by general physicians and dermatologists, it is believed the actual figure is closer to 100,000 cases a year. In fact, malignant melanoma is increasing worldwide, faster than any other cancer. One of the latest figures predicts 1 in 70 Americans will develop melanoma at some time in their lives, and by the year 2010, the melanoma risk will rise to 1 in 50. A sobering thought…

No one has discovered a single cause for melanoma, but some factors appear to play a role:

- There is a higher incidence of malignant melanoma in summer climates.
- Many dermatologists believe that excessive sun exposure at an early age, and severe blistering sunburns at any age, will predispose one to malignant melanoma.
- There is a greater frequency in Caucasians versus other races, as a result of the superior ultraviolet screening capacity provided by darker skin.
- People who develop melanoma are likely to have light-colored eyes, light complexions and haircolor, and seem to sunburn easily.
- Although melanomas are uncommon in blacks, they can arise on the more lightly pigmented portions of the skin: the palms, soles, the nail beds, and mucous membranes of the mouth.
- If your parents, children, or siblings have had a melanoma, you have a much greater risk of developing one.
- More melanomas develop on the legs of women than men. This

phenomenon is attributed to the greater exposure to sunlight as a result of women's habit of dress.

- Women taking oral contraceptives run a far greater risk of developing these black cancers.
- Injury may also play a role in the development of melanoma. In the barefooted African Bantu, melanoma of the sole is more prevalent than in those who wear shoes, and in Ugandans the most common site of melanoma is on the sole.

Bleak as this picture is, malignant melanoma can be cured surgically in over 50 percent of cases. The key to success is prompt therapy. However, one can never be certain a melanoma has actually been cured, particularly those tumors that penetrate the lower layers of the skin and subcutaneous tissue, spreading to the lymph glands.

A new vaccine being tested in Canada promises a modicum of encouragement for those with early melanomas. It is still too early for any definitive results, but the medical companies are optimistic.

How do you know whether to worry about existing moles? Suspect a mole if it had undergone any change in size, shape, color, or texture. The **A, B, C, D danger signs of melanoma** are as follows:

A. Asymmetry. If one half of a mole is unlike the other half.
B. Border irregularity. A scalloped or poorly circumscribed border should alert one.
C. Color varies from one area to another. Look for shades of red, white, or blue. Black is suspicious.
D. Diameter is larger than a quarter of an inch.

Moles that itch, crust, bleed, change texture or ulcerate also point to a possible malignant change. See your physician at once if you notice any of these changes. He or she will more than likely recommend surgical excision of the worrisome mole followed by microscopic analysis of the tissue.

For more information on melanoma, log on to:
www.melanoma.com or www.aad.org
or phone: 1-888-462-DERM x22

Recap

- Evidence from many sources suggests a steadily rising incidence of malignant melanoma in the past few decades accompanied by a rising death rate.
- Unlike the other cancers of the skin, the melanoma has a striking tendency to spread to other parts of the body.
- If your parents, children, or siblings have had a melanoma, you have a much greater risk of developing one.

DIMPLE WARTS

Dimple warts are benign (friendly) skin tumors in the top layers of the skin caused by a virus, the largest of all true viruses known to cause human disease. The scientific name for these growths is molluscum contagiosum. While similar to the common wart, they are caused by a different virus.

These warts occur most frequently in children and young adults. They do not itch, hurt, or burn, but they are highly contagious. They can spread indirectly (through towels, washcloths, and similar items) or directly from person to person as on wrestling mats and in swimming pools. Epidemics of these viral tumors are common among children and adolescents in schools, orphanages, and other institutions. In sexually active people it is considered a sexually transmitted disease.

Molluscum contagiosum are more common in tropical climates, as warmth and humidity tend to favor the growth of the virus, and in people who are immunocompromised such as those with AIDS.

It usually takes about six weeks from the time of contact or exposure until the disease appears. The virus enters the skin through small injuries, scratches, insect bites, or puncture wounds. The tumors usually begin as pinhead-sized elevations that gradually enlarge to the size of a small pea. They may persist for years but usually stop growing once they reach this size.

The elevations—known as nodules—are smooth, dome-shaped, and either waxy or pearly in appearance. Older molluscums usually develop a dimple resembling a belly button (hence the name: dimple wart). The lesions are often confined to the abdomen, thighs, pubic area, and genitals, but can occur on any portion of the skin surface. When they occur on the eyelids of young children, they are very difficult to eradicate by surgical means. Non-sexual transmission of the condition is often seen in wrestlers.

When squeezed, dimple warts discharge a milky-white, curd-like substance. Left untreated, they usually disappear by themselves after months or years without leaving scars. Since they are contagious, however, there are some measures you should take.

Avoid touching the people you know have the virus, and practice good hygiene. Keep clean! A dermatologist can eradicate them quickly and almost painlessly by any of a variety of methods. One popular technique is to freeze them off with liquid nitrogen. They also can be burned off (cauterized) under local anesthesia, scraped off with a small curette (actually a "round knife"), or destroyed with various chemicals. All of these procedures are safe and effective.

For further information about dimple warts, log on to
www.aad.org
or phone: 1-888-462-DERM x22

Recap

• Dimple warts are benign (friendly) skin tumors in the top layers of the skin caused by a virus, the largest of all true viruses known to cause human disease.

• These dimple warts occur most frequently in children and young adults. They do not itch, hurt, or burn, but they are highly contagious.

• Molluscum contagiosum can spread indirectly (through towels, washcloths, and similar items) or directly between people, as on wrestling mats and in swimming pools.

VASCULAR BIRTHMARKS

Many babies—about ten percent—are born with what are commonly called "birthmarks." These benign lesions are usually made up of blood vessels that collect in certain parts of the skin. They can be raised or flat; they can be pink or red or bluish. No one knows why they appear nor can anyone predict where they will appear. We do know they are not inherited.

One of the most common vascular birthmarks is called the "port-wine stain," technically known as "nevus flammeus." This is a flat, reddish-purple mark that appears most often on the back of the neck and on the face. Mikhail Gorbachev, the former President of the Soviet Union, has a very large, identifiable port-wine stain over his scalp. When they are small, and located over the forehead or eyelids, they are sometimes called "angel's kisses." When they are located over the back of the neck—about 25 percent of people have this type of birthmark—the slang is "stork bites." These birthmarks are harmless and require no treatment. The "angel's kisses" usually disappear by the age of two or three; the "stork bites" last into adulthood and often never fade away. If the "port-wine stains" are large, early laser therapy intervention is recommended.

Hemangiomas, the most common tumors of infancy, are familiar vascular birthmarks. About 30 percent of all hemangiomas are visible at birth; the remaining 70 percent become visible within the first few weeks of life. No one knows why hemangiomas occur. They are not hereditary.

Hemangiomas are usually divided into two types: the strawberry hemangioma—slightly raised and bright red because the blood vessels are very close to the skin surface; and the cavernous hemangioma—bluish because the abnormal blood vessels are deeper under the skin. They are more common in female and in premature babies. They can vary in size from small and innocuous to large and deforming, but are usually less than 3 inches in diameter. More than 80 percent occur in the head and neck region. They can grow for up to 2 years and then begin to turn white and involute.

If your baby has a birthmark, it's important to have a dermatologist evaluate it. There are several treatments available for these cosmetic blights, the latest being the new variety of lasers. If the lesions are large, corrective surgery is an option.

For further information about vascular birthmarks, log on to:
www.aad.org
or phone: 1-888-462-DERM x22

Recap

- Vascular birthmarks are not inherited.
- If your baby has a birthmark, it's important to have a dermatologist evaluate it.

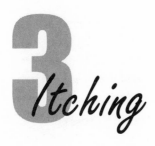

Itching

"Scratching is one of nature's sweetest gratifications of nature, and as ready at hand as any."

—Montaigne

Itching, simply stated, is the urge to scratch. The medical term for itching is pruritus. It is a common, everyday experience ranging from a simple, fleeting annoyance (a mosquito bite) to the intense, distressing, unrelieved torment (the itch of scabies) that can result in sleepless nights.

Why do people itch? Let me try to explain.

We know that the sensations of pain and itch are carried to the brain by the same nerve fibers, and we know that pain and itching points have similar distribution on the surface of the skin. We also know that it's possible, by varying the intensity of a stimulus (chemical, electrical, or physical) to cause either pain or itching on a certain portion of the skin.

So, a better way of understanding this complex sensation is to consider an itch a sub-threshold pain, or better still, a pain that doesn't hurt. The difference is that an itch occurs only in the skin, while actual pain arises from deeper structures. And while itching leads to the urge to scratch, pain leads to withdrawal from the stimulus.

Have you ever bruised, scraped, or skinned your knee or

elbow? Have you ever suffered from moderately severe sunburn? If you have, you may remember that at first there were varying degrees of pain. When the bruise, scrape, or burn began to heal, this pain was gradually transformed into an itch—a so-called "healing" itch: a peculiar sensation in the skin that produces a desire to scratch.

Commonly experienced, unpredictable, and poorly understood, itching is the symptom that most frequently prompts a visit to the dermatologist.

Different people experience, interpret, and tolerate itching in different degrees. One person's itch might be another person's tickle; one person's stinging itch can be another person's pain. If you have a high itch threshold, a transient mosquito bite or a brush with a poison ivy plant will rarely bother you. Less fortunate people will itch unmercifully at the least provocation, such as a mild allergy to nickel earrings or a simple rash from a leather watchband. No one knows why.

Many years ago scientists thought that the basic cause of itching was the release of a chemical substance called histamine. We now know that itching can be caused by a breakdown of various tissue proteins, and precipitated by a variety of stimuli, such as the following:

- Chemical: plants (poison ivy), drugs (aspirin, penicillin), foods (berries, seafood, nuts), metals (nickel, chromium); cosmetics, paints and sprays.
- Physical: heat, cold, pressure, and friction.
- Infestations: lice, mites (scabies), insect bites and stings.
- Germs: athlete's foot, cold sores, impetigo.
- Skin disorders: eczema, allergy rashes, hives, lichen planus, dry skin.
- Psychogenic: anxiety, tension, and emotional stress.
- Systemic disease: diabetes and other hormonal disorders, liver and kidney problems, malignant diseases.
- Blood disorders: leukemias, Hodgkin's disease.

What do you do when you itch? You scratch…naturally.

Why does scratching relieve itching? Again, no one really knows. It may be that by scratching or rubbing you are substituting the sensation of pain for that of itching. Or, it may be that by scratching you damage the nerve fibers that cause the itching. Scratching, while it provides temporary relief, can actually cause more harm than good. It can lead to secondary infection, which may require internal antibiotic therapy.

What *should* you do when you itch?

The most important thing to do is determine, if you can, why you began to itch in the first place. If you do not have a clue and your itch persists, see a dermatologist.

What you can do to relieve itching depends, of course, on the cause. No single therapy is effective for every itch. In addition to providing symptomatic relief, most treatments are aimed at eliminating the underlying cause.

For symptomatic relief of mild to moderate itching—regardless of the cause—you can try several over-the-counter remedies:

- Any of the over-the-counter hydrocortisone creams for localized itchy areas, or
- Calamine Lotion, Sarna Lotion, Aveeno Anti-Itch Lotion, or Caladryl if the rash is more extensive. Apply to the itchy areas every 3 or 4 hours.
- Over-the-counter oral antihistamines. (Take according to the directions on the package.)
- If the itching is fairly generalized, take soothing baths using a therapeutic baths preparation such as Aveeno Oatmeal Bath.

If your itching is severe, persistent, and unrelieved by over-the-counter measures, consult with a dermatologist. It may be the initial manifestation of a relatively serious underlying systemic disease and not a simple itch after all.

For further information about itching, log on to: www.aad.org
1-888-462-DERM x22

Recap

- Itching is a common, everyday experience ranging from a simple, fleeting annoyance to intense, distressing, unrelieved torment that can result in sleepless nights.
- Commonly experienced, unpredictable, and poorly understood, itching is the symptom that most frequently prompts a person to visit a dermatologist.

We have already examined most of the familiar skin conditions. There are literally hundreds more. Following, are common and annoying disorders of the skin and mucous membranes.

4 Other Skin Ailments

CANKER SORES

Canker sores are painful ulcerations in the mouth affecting about 25 percent of the population. The medical term for this baffling condition is aphthous stomatitis—but these sores by any other name are just as painful.

Many people confuse canker sores with cold sores. A virus causes cold sores. But we know little about what causes canker sores and even less about what cures them. Nor do we know what prevents them. We *do* know that they are not contagious, they are more common in women, they are not hereditary, and they do not cause cancer.

Canker sores develop as small blisters in the mouth, singly or in groups, which usually go unnoticed. These blisters break, and small, round, shallow ulcers develop. The ulcers gradually enlarge and become yellow and shiny with bright red borders. They can be exquisitely tender and painful—so painful sometimes that it can disrupt eating.

Canker sores can be found anywhere in the mouth: the inside of the cheeks, the lips, sides of the tongue, the floor of the mouth, the gums, and the palate. They heal by themselves in about two weeks without leaving scars. Unfortunately, however, they tend to recur. Some people develop them every few weeks, others every few months, and some unlucky few are never without them.

Although no one knows what causes these painful mouth sores, many of the following triggering factors have been suspected:

- Poor dental hygiene. Inadequate and improper brushing and flossing may give rise to these painful ulcerations.
- Injury caused by stiff toothbrushes, poorly fitting dentures, as well as certain denture materials have been known to provoke canker sores.
- Foods such as chocolate, citrus fruits, spices, milk, cola drinks, and nuts, especially English walnuts, can activate canker sores in susceptible people.
- Allergies to drugs. Some common offenders are aspirin, antibiotics, sulfa drugs, and chemotherapeutic agents to treat cancer.
- Illness accompanied by fever.
- Menstruation.
- Fatigue, emotional stress and tension.
- Viruses (similar to the viral infection responsible for cold sores).
- Bacteria.
- Many patients—and other dermatologists—have told me that shortly after they gave up smoking, they began to develop canker sores, and when they started to smoke again the sores disappeared never to return. However, I do not recommend smoking to alleviate or prevent canker sores!

If you have recurrent canker sores the following general measures may prevent attacks:
- Keep your mouth clean.
- Avoid all kinds of nuts and any foods you suspect might be triggering factors.
- Stop chewing gum, and discontinue mouthwashes.
- If you are using fluoridated toothpaste, especially one with Tartar Control (and who isn't?), switch to a nonfluoridated brand. Tom's Toothpaste is one, but make sure you get the one without fluoride. Or substitute salt or baking soda.
- If they appear before your menstrual period, take an antihistamine daily, beginning a week or ten days prior to it.

If none of these measures help, consult a dermatologist or dentist. Either one may be able to pinpoint the cause of your sores and suggest additional treatment.

Theories on treating an existing attack of canker sores are almost as varied as the suspected causes. Among the many cures that dermatologists and dentists recommend are dental ointments containing a "relative" of cortisone; painting the sores with silver nitrate solution; injecting a cortisone-like drug beneath the ulcers; and taking lozenges.

There is, however, only one proven reliable method of relieving the pain due to canker sores: using mouthwashes or "compresses" with tetracycline. Tetracycline is a prescription antibiotic. This treatment involves emptying a 250-milligram capsule (not tablet) of tetracycline into one to two ounces of warm water and shaking it up very well. (Tetracycline powder cannot be dissolved in water but forms a suspension when shaken.) Swish this solution around in your mouth for five or ten minutes every two or three hours or soak wads of cotton in it and apply to the sores. Both methods should give prompt relief. (Tetracycline syrup does not give the same, if any, relief of these painful sores. Only the powdered suspension can do it.)

For those who are plagued with recurrent canker sores, I recommend eating at least four tablespoonfuls of unflavored yogurt every day and discontinuing all nuts. If you do this daily, you may never experience a canker sore again.

For further information about canker sores, log on to www.aad.org
or www.familydoctor.org/handouts/613.html
1-888-462-DERM x22

Recap

- Canker sores—aphthous stomatitis—are painful ulcerations in the mouth affecting about twenty-five percent of the population.
- Canker sores can be found anywhere in the mouth: the inside of the cheeks, the lips, sides of the tongue, the floor of the mouth, the gums, and the palate.
- Some people develop canker sores every few weeks, others every few months, and some unlucky few are never without them.

DIAPER RASH AND PRICKLY HEAT

Diaper Rash

Diaper rash, the bane of young mothers, the frustration of young fathers, and often the challenge of seasoned pediatricians, is a very common skin ailment. Beginning for the most part between the ages of two and four months, this itchy, burning, painful, nasty-looking rash can result in restlessness, irritability, and sleep interruption. It can persist for months or until your child outgrows diapers.

Also known as napkin or diaper dermatitis, diaper rash is any eruption on an infant's buttocks, genital and anal areas, lower abdomen, and upper thighs. Although the problem is usually a minor one, it can, when ignored, lead to widespread infection, necessitating vigorous and prolonged treatment.

In its early and simple form, diaper rash is characterized by redness or chafing of the skin that touches the diaper. When left untreated small pimples, called papules, and water blisters, called vesicles, develop. This can progress to oozing, sogginess in the skin folds and, in severe cases, open sores. The sharp, pungent odor of ammonia usually accompanies this rash.

The villain in all cases of diaper rash is, sad to say, the diaper. Babies do not, and cannot, develop diaper rash if they do not wear diapers! In our society, however, it is *de rigueur* for our infants to sport diapers: cloth, synthetic, treated, odor preventing, and a host of other types and styles. Most Greek babies—primarily those brought up on the smaller islands—do not develop diaper rash because they are regularly cleansed by their mothers who cradle them in their left arm while washing away the urine and soiling under a stream of warm tap water.

Other causes of diaper rash include rubber or plastic pants that prevent the skin from "breathing." This can be further aggravated by the rough edges of these pants, as well as by tightly pinned diapers.

Frequent loose stools with their noxious intestinal enzymes can irritate the delicate diaper area, especially when these stools have not been completely removed by cleaning. Other causes of irritation include harsh soaps for cleaning the skin; strong detergents, antiseptic rinses, perfumed fabric softeners, assorted baby oils, salves, ointments, and other chemical irritants.

High humidity also contributes to diaper rash, as it causes the skin and skin folds to become waterlogged. This creates an inflammation around the sweat pores and prevents the normal flow of perspiration, thus lowering the resistance of the skin to infection. The normal, usually "friendly" and harmless germs, such as bacteria and fungi, then begin to thrive, setting up housekeeping in these trapped fluids. They become "unfriendly" and harmful.

Although the situation often seems dismal, there are some positive steps you can take to prevent and treat diaper rash. Here are a few suggestions for prevention:

- Use soft, cotton diapers.
- Change diapers as soon as they are soiled *and* at regular intervals. Newborns urinate more than 20 times a day and one-year-olds average six or seven times a day. Therefore, be on the alert and learn to anticipate.
- Use plastic and rubber pants only sparingly and for short periods of time, such as for party occasions. Never use them at night.
- Following each diaper change, clean the diaper area thoroughly but gently with a mild cleanser, such as Cetaphil Cleanser, to remove all bacterial and fecal contamination. Pay careful attention to the skin folds. These folds should be washed gently and then rinsed thoroughly to make certain that all the cleanser is completely removed.
- Dry the skin and the skin folds thoroughly.
- Use a medicated cornstarch-based powder two or three times daily to keep the affected areas dry.
- Wash diapers in mild soap or detergent. Make sure they are carefully and painstakingly rinsed.
- Don't use the perfumed fabric softener pads for clothes dryers. Even the non-perfumed varieties have a softening agent that may also be responsible for aggravating diaper rash.
- Dress your child in clothing that is porous enough to allow good air circulation.
- Keep air in the child's room cool and dry.
- Encourage early training in regular toilet habits.

If your child is already suffering from diaper rash, the following steps can help clear it up and forestall further irritation, inflammation, and infection:

- Stop all previous medication.
- Discontinue plastic and rubber pants.
- Never use soap when the skin is inflamed.
- Apply wet dressings, compresses, or 15-minute baths using Burow's Solution (two Bluboro or Dome-Boro or Pedi-Boro packets dissolved in one quart of warm water) every three or four hours to soothe and cool the inflamed areas.
- Allow the affected areas to "breathe." Air is a marvelous healing agent. I strongly recommend that you permit infants and children with diaper rash to lie about and run around naked for several hours a day! Remember: your child cannot develop a diaper rash if he or she doesn't wear diapers.

During the acute stage of diaper rash, I urge that you discontinue *all* diapers during the day. Use a double layer of soft, cotton diapers, very loosely pinned, at night. Never use plastic or rubber pants at any time.

When the inflammation, oozing, and sogginess have begun to clear, use a soothing and protective preparation such as Zinc Oxide Ointment at night. Finally, when the affected areas have adequately healed and the child is more comfortable, use soft cotton diapers again.

Be especially careful and conscientious, change the sheets as often as necessary, wash the soiled areas gently but thoroughly, and reapply the Zinc Oxide Ointment after each soiling.

Prickly Heat

Prickly heat is a common disorder of the sweat apparatus. It arises when the free flow of sweat to the surface of the skin is obstructed. The medical term for this condition is miliaria.

Sweat is produced by the more than 2 million sweat glands in the skin. Under normal conditions, it flows out smoothly and uninterrupted to the skin surface through tiny sweat ducts. If the sweat is heavy and prolonged, it can clog the ducts and become trapped. This trapped sweat, unable to reach the skin surface, breaks through the walls of the ducts. The result is an inflammation of the skin known as prickly heat, or heat rash.

While prickly heat can materialize at any age, there is a tendency for it to occur more commonly in infants for two reasons: the relatively small size of the sweat ducts encourages closing of the pores thereby favoring sweat retention, and parent's overprotection of the infant from the cold contributes to the warmth and humidity in which heat rash flourishes.

Prickly heat often appears suddenly and takes the form of numerous, tiny, reddish pimples and water blisters scattered in the creases of the neck, under the chin, in the armpits, and on the chest, back, abdomen, and buttocks. Recurrent crops may continue indefinitely and can cause restlessness and irritability, as well as burning and prickling sensations.

Prickly heat can result from any condition that encourages profuse and prolonged sweating along with inadequate evaporation of the sweat. The offender can be an excessively hot and humid climate or a fever. Indeed, persistent and extensive cases of heat rash are most common in tropical climes. Aggravated by obesity and tightly fitting garments, prickly heat usually clears up on its own, and only rarely do secondary bacterial and fungal infections materialize. While it lasts, however, it can be very distressing, particularly for young children.

Fortunately, there are some simple and effective methods to prevent or treat prickly heat. The primary concern is to keep the *skin* cool and dry. This is easy: keep the *air* cool and dry. Other helpful suggestions include the following:

- Use an air-conditioner or fan to reduce the temperature and humidity.
- Maintain adequate room ventilation to encourage the evaporation of sweat.
- Dress your child in loose-fitting, lightweight cotton clothing and limit physical activity in hot, humid weather.

If prickly heat has already taken place, try the following treatment:

- Apply soothing, drying lotions such as plain calamine lotion.
- Use a cornstarch-based dusting powder.
- If possible, allow the afflicted child to lie about the house naked.
- Wash with a cleanser, such as Cetaphil Cleanser, and never use greases or ointments that will further clog the sweat ducts.
- During the acute phase of prickly heat, give the child lukewarm baths, preferably with Linit Starch or Aveeno Bath Regular Formula.

Of course, the main answer to prickly heat is to stay cool!

For further information about diaper rash, log on to www.aad.org
or www.familydoctor.org/healthfacts/051
1-888-462-DERM x22

Recap

- Diaper rash is any eruption on an infant's buttocks, genital and anal areas, lower abdomen, and upper thighs that manifests itself during the diaper-wearing stage.
- During the acute stage of diaper rash, discontinue *all* diapers during the day. Use a double layer of soft, cotton diapers, very loosely pinned, at night. Never use plastic or rubber pants at any time.
- Prickly heat can result from any condition that encourages profuse and prolonged sweating along with inadequate evaporation of the sweat. The offender can be an excessively hot and humid climate or a fever.

ADVERSE DRUG REACTIONS ON THE SKIN

"Any rash can be due to any drug."

It is an inescapable truth that more and more people—primarily the older population—are increasing their intake of over-the-counter and prescription medications. New drugs for all types of disorders—high blood pressure, stomach ulcers, diabetes, high cholesterol, etc.—are appearing in the medical marketplace almost daily. And there are more than 1,800 new drugs in the pipeline at any one time.

Unfortunately, more and more adverse drug reactions, primarily by the skin and hair, have arisen from many of these medications.

Who, for example, does not take aspirin? Tylenol? Advil or Motrin? Who is not treated with an antibiotic when suffering from some bacterial or viral infection? How many of you are being treated with a beta-blocker? An ACE-inhibitor? An antidepressant? A cholesterol-lowering drug? A nonsteroidal anti-inflammatory drug for arthritis or aches and pains? Celebrex? Vioxx? There is not a medication in the marketplace that cannot give rise to some form of drug reaction in certain unfortunate sensitive individuals.

The incidence of advance drug reactions increases with age. The chances of an adverse drug reaction is three times greater for older persons than for younger adults, and forty percent of people who suffer an adverse reaction are over age sixty.

It has been documented that more than 100,000 hospitalized patients die from some adverse drug reaction every year. Nearly 3 billion prescriptions are filled each year; more than 300,000 over-the-counter medicines are also available; and over $77 billion dollars are spent each year as a result of drug reactions due to these medications.

The most common form of drug eruption is a measles-like form of rash called an exanthem. Exanthems can be a result of a myriad number of drugs, primarily aspirin, penicillin and its derivatives such as ampicillin and amoxicillin, and a host of other antibacterial agents such as sulfa drugs. Almost one-quarter of all drug reactions on the skin are the result of these antibacterial agents. It is not common knowledge that those people who are allergic to sulfa drugs may also be allergic to medications prescribed for high blood pressure almost all of which contain some form of thiazide.

Thiazide contains sulfa! So do most oral antidiabetic medications. In addition, many common products are sulfa-based. Saccharin and cyclamates are sulfa drugs, so that if you are allergic to sulfa, you might break out in a rash from sweeteners containing saccharin or cyclamates. (Aspartame, a constituent of Equal or Nutrasweet, is an exception.)

There are also many acne medications, vaginal creams, burn medicines, and eye drops (the newest is Trusopt) that are sulfa based. Celebrex, used for painful arthritis, is also a sulfa drug! Make sure that your doctor knows if you are allergic to sulfa drugs. (Not sulfur, which is an entirely different entity.)

Many people develop itchy rashes when exposed to the sun or to sunbeds after having taken a medication. These are known as photosensitive reactions. They are extremely common after taking sulfa drugs. Exanthems, hives, and severe itching can develop from the combination of these medications and the sun. Oral medications taken for fungous infections (griseofulvin) and those being prescribed for the treatment of many urinary tract infections (Gantrisin and Macrodantin to name a couple) are often responsible for severe, generalized itchy skin. So are the latest "floxin" drugs: Floxin, Levaquin, Zagam, Tequin, Avelox, Cipro, and other quinolone drugs, which can occasion very severe reactions, some leading to death. These reactions, by the way, can develop with or without exposure to the sun's rays.

Have you been losing hair lately? Perhaps you have been taking a beta-blocker or, if you are a woman, you might be taking hormones such as Provera or other progesterone-containing medication for PMS or for menopausal symptoms. These and other drugs, including Tylenol, Motrin, Advil, birth control pills, antidepressants and tranquilizers, anti-ulcer drugs (Tagamet and Zantac), can all bring about hair loss, particularly in women. So do Inderal and a few dozen other prescription and over-the-counter medications. In addition, almost all chemotherapeutic agents can cause reversible hair loss in both men and women.

Muscle pains and aches have been reported from taking any of the so-called "statins:" the lipid-lowering medications such as Lipitor, Pravachol, Zocor, Mevacor, and others.

Many drugs cause metallic taste, dry mouth, itching, swollen gums, depression, ringing in the ears, and dozens of other symptoms.

Blisters on the skin or in the mouth are often adverse effects of various medications including phenobarbital, sulfa drugs, betablockers, ACE-inhibitors, and gold compounds. Many drugs are responsible for excessive pigmentation of the skin. Some of these are oral contraceptives, antibiotics (notably minocycline), and various chemotherapeutic drugs—those used to treat a variety of cancers.

If you are taking any type of medication, and if you find that you have either a rash or hair loss or itching or some other abnormal symptom, check with your physician. It may all be a result of the drug you have been taking.

For further information about drug eruptions, log on to
www.aad.org
or www.familydoctor.org/handouts/231.html
1-888-462-DERM x22

Recap

- The most common form of drug eruption is a measles-like form of rash called an exanthem. Exanthems can be a result of a myriad number of drugs, primarily aspirin and penicillin.
- Many people develop itchy rashes when, after having taken a medication, they had been exposed to the sun or to sunbeds. These are known as photosensitive reactions and are extremely common after taking sulfa drugs.
- People who are allergic to sulfa drugs may also be allergic to medications prescribed for high blood pressure almost all of which contain some form of thiazide. Thiazides contain sulfa!

FROSTBITE

"Men leave arms and legs behind, severed by the frost, and the cruel cold cuts off the limbs already broken."
—Silius Italica, *Punica,* III, 552

Frostbite—the sharp, painful sensations that result from the freezing and thawing of the skin. It is a severe cold injury that, in many ways, resembles the burn you get when you touch something hot. Press an ice cube on your cheeks for a few seconds. Burns, doesn't it? If you were to leave it there for a few minutes, you would develop a painful blister.

Whether exposure to cold will result in frostbite depends on many factors, including the temperature, the wind-chill factor, how long you're exposed, and what you're wearing. People's tolerance to cold varies as well. There are several conditions that reduce one's tolerance: poor circulation, poor general health, poor nutrition, fatigue, injury, immobility of an extremity, and contact with metals.

The areas of the body most vulnerable to the effects of frostbite are the feet and toes, the tip of the nose, the rims and lobes of the ears, and the tips of the fingers.

How do you recognize frostbite? In its mildest form, known as frost nip, the skin suddenly turns pale due to the constriction of blood vessels. This is the body's method of conserving heat by diverting the blood to the vital internal organs. This skin pallor is accompanied by tingling. Burning and pain follow, and the skin turns whitish or slightly yellow.

If the freezing continues, it affects the deeper tissues. The pain disappears and areas affected become numb. (Disappearance of pain is a warning sign of imminent danger!) The affected skin then becomes waxy white. Severe and lengthy exposure to cold can injure deeper tissues, such as muscles, tendons, nerves, and bones. Children who suffer severe cases of frostbitten fingers often end up with small hands as adults.

If you develop frostbite, see your doctor at once. *Do not* treat it with ice, ice water, or snow. This "cold" treatment can actually kill the tissue. And do not move any skin that is frozen—movement will result in severe damage. Also, don't smoke or drink alcohol.

The best method to treat frostbite—the one that your doctor will probably recommend—is to restore the normal temperature of the skin by *rapidly* rewarming the frostbitten area. Immerse the affected part in a water bath at a temperature of 104° to 110° F (40° to 44° C). Better yet, use a whirlpool bath. Make sure the temperature does not exceed 110° F because your skin does not have any sensation, and you could produce a burn at higher temperatures. Do not use local, dry heat. And do not move the frozen skin. This treatment may produce more pain, more redness and swelling, and bigger blisters than gradual rewarming, but it promotes faster healing, reduces tissue loss, and prevents complications, such as infection, ulceration, gangrene, and even loss of a limb.

During the thawing process, blisters will develop. These blisters may persist for weeks, and the newly formed skin may be tender for months. In most cases of mild to moderate frostbite, complete healing will usually take place in a week or two.

To guard against frostbite, dress normally and protect those parts that are most susceptible to cold. When the temperature falls and the wind is howling, causing the chill factor to drop to arctic levels, protect those delicate sensitive areas: the fingertips with warm gloves or mittens; the ears with muffs or flaps; and the nose with a ski mask. The feet should be enclosed in thick, loose-fitting, lined boots that can accommodate thick socks. Protect the rest of the body with thermal underwear, long johns, turtleneck sweaters, scarves, and fur-lined coats. The ideal fabric for outdoor wear is one that traps a lot of air. Loosely woven bulky wool or acrylic, Thinsulate, Holowfil, Goretex and PolarGuard all fill this guideline.

Keep up your general health and avoid fatigue.

For further information about frostbite, log on to:
www.aad.org
1-888-462-DERM x22

Recap

- Whether exposure to cold will result in frostbite depends on many factors, including the temperature, the wind-chill factor, how long you're exposed, and what you're wearing.
- The areas of the body most vulnerable to the effects of frostbite are the feet and toes, the tip of the nose, the rims and lobes of the ears, and the tips of the fingers.
- If you develop frostbite, see your doctor at once. *Do not* treat it with ice, ice water, or snow. This "cold" treatment can actually kill the tissue.

ICHTHYOSIS

Ichthyosis, or "fishskin disease," is a relatively uncommon, hereditary abnormality of the skin that afflicts more than one million Americans. Derived from the Greek word *ichthys* (fish), the term ichthyosis refers to the fish-scale appearance of the skin. The

"Alligator Man," "Lizard Woman" and "Porcupine Man" of old-time circus sideshows were victims of ichthyosis.

Rather than a single disease entity, ichthyosis represents a family of related diseases. There are four distinct types of these coarse, rough, and scaly skin disorders all of which are characterized by an increase in the thickness of the upper layers of the skin. It is caused by a genetic defect that can be either inherited or spontaneous. It is not due to germs or viruses and is, therefore, not contagious.

Brought about by abnormalities in either protein or fat metabolism, these diseases are a result of either an excessive production of skin cells, or as a consequence of increased "stickiness" of the uppermost layer of the skin—the horny layer—which occasions an impairment in the normal shedding process. The result is dry, thickened skin that shrinks and cracks.

(The upper layer of the skin—the epidermis—is constantly regenerating itself: all its cells turn themselves over about every 28 days. Dead cells slough off as new ones push up in a perpetual and lifelong process of cell division. It takes about two weeks for the newborn cells to make their way to the outermost layer of the epidermis, where they remain, as dead and dying cells, for another two weeks until they are cast off. See the chapter on Dandruff, page 148.)

The two most prevalent types of ichthyosis are ichthyosis vulgaris and X-linked ichthyosis. In both types, the normal shedding process is retarded.

ICHTHYOSIS VULGARIS

The most common—or "vulgar"—type of ichthyosis, known appropriately as ichthyosis vulgaris, develops after the first three months of life and affects about one in every 300 people. It is inherited, may affect several members of a family, and is characterized by fine, white, branny scaling which appears most prominently over the trunk and outside surfaces of the arms and legs. The inside of the elbow and knee areas—the flexures—are not involved, but the palms and soles are often thickened. There is usually no itching or burning or other subjective symptoms; and while the chief complaints of this fishlike, scaly disorder are often only cosmetic in nature, there are other considerations that must be kept in mind.

Children with this condition suffer physical and psychological problems. The skin, which cannot hold moisture, can become tight and stiff; severely limiting the child's ability to play like other children. Even simple tasks can, on occasion, be painful.

Ichthyosis vulgaris improves with age and with warm, moist surroundings. It is often associated with some form of allergy—eczema, hay fever, or asthma—and with dry skin of the palms and heels, that is intensified in cold, dry weather.

X-LINKED ICHTHYOSIS

The second most common type of inherited scaly skin is called X-linked ichthyosis. This more severe variety affects about one in 4,000 males and is transmitted to sons by unaffected mothers. As in ichthyosis vulgaris, this variant results from retarded shedding of the uppermost layers of the skin.

Characterized by early onset—from birth until about one year—and generalized involvement, this condition displays large, coarse, adherent, "stuck-on" scales over the neck, trunk, buttocks, and outer portions of the extremities. When the neck is affected, it invariably has an unwashed appearance. X-linked ichthyosis becomes increasingly severe with the passage of time.

While there is no cure for ichthyosis, various therapies can greatly improve the appearance of the skin and relieve the excessive dryness and scaling. The goal of therapy is to keep the scales from building up and to retain moisture in the upper layers of the skin.

A prescription cream—Lac-Hydrin Cream 12%—has offered genuine relief in many sufferers for the past few years. Some of the over-the-counter alpha-hydroxy acids have also provided modest improvements. Use a mild cleanser, such as Cetaphil Cleanser, when cleaning the skin.

If the person lives in a warm, humid environment, little treatment is required for either type of ichthyosis just described. Keeping the relative humidity levels above 60 percent is vital.

For further information about ichthyosis, contact:
F.I.R.S.T.
(Foundation for Ichthyosis & Related Skin Types)
650 N. Cannon Avenue—Suite 17
Lansdale, PA 19446
800-545-3286; 215-631-1411
E-mail: focus@scalyskin.org
www.scalyskin.org
In addition, there is a National Registry for Ichthyosis
University of Washington Dermatology
Box 356524—Seattle, WA 98195-65524
800-595-1265
E-mail: ichreg@u.washington.edu

Recap

- Ichthyosis is caused by a genetic defect that can be either inherited or spontaneous. It is not due to germs or viruses and is, therefore, not contagious.
- The most common—or "vulgar"—type of ichthyosis, known appropriately as ichthyosis vulgaris, develops after the first three months of life and affects about one in every 300 people.
- While there is no cure for ichthyosis, various therapies can greatly improve the appearance of the skin and relieve the excessive dryness and scaling. The goal of therapy is to keep the scales from building up and to retain moisture in the upper layers of the skin.

IMPETIGO

Impetigo is a highly contagious, unsightly skin infection caused by the streptococcus and staphylococcus bacteria. The medical term for this condition, appropriately, is impetigo contagiosa.

Impetigo appears as thick, stuck-on, honey-colored crusts usually around the nostrils and mouth, although any portion of the skin surface may be affected. It occurs primarily in children, but adults can fall victim, too, usually by direct contact with infected children

Impetigo begins on damaged skin, when the outer protective layers are injured and the normal resistance of the skin is lowered. This damage can be a result of cuts, bruises, insect bites, or other skin diseases, such as chicken pox, cold sores, or acne. Healthy skin seems to act as a barrier to suppress these harmful bacteria.

The mouth and nose, which suffer constant rubbing and wiping, are the prime areas on which impetigo begins. The infectious germs are carried to other parts of the body by dirty fingers and fingernails, as well as unclean towels, utensils, and clothing. These germs can spread to other people who have direct contact with infected persons, especially through kissing, wrestling, or other such contact sports.

Once impetigo takes hold, it spreads very easily, even to normal healthy skin, and may last for several weeks. If not controlled it can lead to internal infections accompanied by fever, fatigue, and swollen lymph glands.

Those infected with impetigo should seek prompt medical attention. A doctor's care can control its spread, especially to other members of the family and friends, and possibly prevent the serious internal complications, such as kidney infections that may arise.

Treatment consists of gently removing the crusts and thoroughly cleansing the affected areas four times daily with a good antibacterial soap like *Dial* or *Safeguard*. If the crusts stick stubbornly to the underlying skin, you may need to apply warm water compresses to lift them off.

After each thorough washing, rub in an antibiotic ointment, such as *Polysporin*. (I do not recommend any ointments that have neomycin in them, such as *Neosporin*, as they are great sensitizing agents and can cause allergic rashes.) *Do not cover the area with bandages or gauze.* Exposure to air will help kill many types of germs and speed the healing process.

If the condition appears extensive and severe, see your physician.

The following are some additional measures that help eliminate impetigo and prevent its spread:

- Wash hands thoroughly and frequently with an antibacterial soap.
- Avoid touching sores as infection can spread easily to other parts of your body.
- Keep fingernails trimmed and scrupulously clean at all times.
- Change your towels daily.

- Since impetigo is contagious, avoid close contact with friends and relatives, and keep the children home during the acute, crusted stage of the disease.
- Continue treatment for seven to ten days after all the crusts are gone.

If the lesions persist after several days of treatment, contact your physician for further treatment. This treatment may include an oral antibiotic or a penicillin injection.

For further information about impetigo, log on to www.aad.org
1-888-462-DERM x22

Recap

- Impetigo is a highly contagious, unsightly skin infection caused by the streptococcus and staphylococcus bacteria.
- Impetigo appears as thick, stuck-on, honey-colored crusts usually around the nostrils and mouth, although any portion of the skin surface may be affected.
- If the lesions persist after several days of treatment, contact your physician for further treatment. This treatment may include an oral antibiotic or a penicillin injection.

INFESTATIONS

While parasites are not considered a major problem for people in the United States, there are two types of similar organisms that have recently have caused virtual epidemics. These organisms—called ectoparasites—are lice and mites.

Infestations with lice (true insects) and mites (insect-like organisms) cause intensely itchy, annoying skin problems. Unless diagnosed and treated properly, these conditions can persist and eventually spread to family members, classmates, and friends.

Lice

Lice are small, wingless insects about one-eighth of an inch in length. They have been around for centuries and have flourished on the persons of both the rich and poor.

Associated with wars and disease in the Middle Ages, lice carry typhus, a disease known to wipe out entire armies. They were extremely prevalent throughout the world until World War II, when DDT almost eradicated this annoying and dread pestilence. However, the ban on DDT as a hazardous substance, along with the increase in social contact and world travel, has contributed to a resurgence of louse infestation.

Today lice have become a major public health problem throughout the world. Aggravated by poor living conditions, lack of personal cleanliness, and overcrowding, this infestation has reached epidemic proportions. Lice are so common in Japan that pediculicides are distributed free in Japanese bathhouses.

The main symptoms of louse infestation—known technically as pediculosis—is a relentless, maddening itch caused by the saliva of the female louse.

There are three kinds of lice affecting three different body areas: head lice, pubic lice, and body lice. Although each type has a different shape, they all feed by biting the skin and sucking the blood.

The adult female louse lays eggs (nits), which she firmly attaches with a glue-like substance to hairs or to fibers of clothing. The eggs hatch in about ten days and reach maturity in about two weeks. Lice have a life span of about one month.

Head Lice

Except for the common cold, head lice is the most frequently occurring communicable disease among children in the United States. Head lice have become especially prevalent in recent years, particularly among school children in urban areas. They make a home in your hair, causing intense itching on your scalp, the back of your neck, and behind your ears. In severe cases they cause swollen lymph glands in your neck. For some reason, head lice are almost never seen in African-American people.

If you look closely, you can see the small, silvery egg cases attached to individual hair shafts. Usually these nits will be close to the scalp—no more than a half-inch from where the hair has emerged. Although they resemble dandruff, they are much more difficult to remove than dandruff flakes because of the sticky, cement-like substance the female louse secretes to attach the nits. Head lice are transmitted by direct contact, by personal items such as combs, brushes, pillowcases, and through clothing like hats, scarves, ribbons, and other head coverings. If one person in a family or classroom has head lice, there is a good possibility that others in the same home or class will have it, too.

If you have head lice, treatment is relatively simple and very effective. Kwell (generic: lindane), a prescription shampoo, will cure a case of head lice in five minutes. One shampoo for five minutes. That's it! There are also non-prescription shampoos—RID, NIX, Pronto, Clear Lice Killing Shampoo—that work about as well.

After shampooing, you may still see eggs attached to the hair shafts, but these are now dead. To get rid of the unsightly but harmless dead nits, apply diluted vinegar (one-half vinegar and one-half water) to your scalp to loosen them. Then back comb with a fine-tooth comb.

Lice that fall off the hair cannot survive longer than 2 or 3 days. Nits, however, can remain viable for up to two weeks off a human host.

To prevent the spread of lice, thoroughly wash all articles of clothing that are suspected of having nits or adult lice.

Pubic Lice ("Crab" Lice)

Pubic lice infestation—commonly called "crabs"—is a highly contagious, sexually transmitted disease. There has been a steady increase in its incidence, with about 2 million new cases a year. For some reason, "crabs" are more common in females between the ages of 15 and 19, and more common in males over the age of twenty.

Usually you get pubic lice through sexual or other close physical contact, but they are also transmitted by sharing a bed or wearing the clothes of an infested person. It's even transmitted—rarely—by toilet seats!

The usual symptom of pubic lice is a maddening itch (especially at night), that scratching doesn't relieve. Like head lice, the nits of

126

pubic lice are usually glued in clusters to the short hair shafts and resemble the flakes of dandruff. Crabs usually set up housekeeping in the pubic region, but during warm, dark, and quiet periods, the adult female lice—along with their eggs—migrate to other short-haired areas of the body—the bellybutton, chest, beard, and men's mustaches, the armpits, and even the eyelashes. Never, however, to the scalp!

The treatment for pubic lice is essentially the same as that for head lice. For lice and nits that have found their way to your eyelashes, apply Johnson's Baby Shampoo or Vaseline with a Q-Tip two or three times daily. This should cure the condition in a few days.

Body Lice

Infestation with body lice is not very common in the United States. Unlike head and crab lice, body lice bite the skin but live in the seams of clothing. Treat the clothing, and the rash will disappear.

Scabies

Scabies is a common and contagious skin disease. It has infested humans for at least 2,500 years. Like lice, it has reached epidemic proportions in the United States. Although scabies is often associated with poverty, crowded living conditions and poor hygiene, there has been a definite increase of the disease in the more affluent. Anybody and everybody can become infested with scabies. It has been estimated that more than 300 million cases of scabies occur worldwide every year.

A mite—a tiny creature, mistakenly referred to as an insect—causes scabies. This mite measures about one seventy-fifth of an inch in length, so small that it is barely visible to the naked eye. These tiny, eight-legged creatures burrow into the skin and spread from one individual to the next through personal and sexual contact. It may take a month before a newly infested person notices the fierce itching characteristic of scabies. Animals, principally dogs, carry a different form of scabies that they can pass on to humans, causing a similar condition.

Scabies is characterized by intense itching due to an allergy to the female mite and the eggs and feces she deposits underneath the upper layers of the skin. This itching becomes more intense at night, when the tiny organisms grow more active, when the person gets overheated, or when they remove their clothing. Often the itching is so severe that it leads to nervousness and loss of sleep. And since the scratching can lead to bleeding, an infested person may have bloodied sheets, pajamas, or underwear.

The scabies mite is most fond of attacking the webs of the fingers, the inner surfaces of the wrists, and the elbows. Other common areas where the mites set up housekeeping are on the chest near the armpits, the area around the bellybutton, the buttocks, the nipples, and the penis. As a rule, infestations above the neck are extremely rare, except in infants and young children where the palms, soles, wrists and buttocks are the most common areas involved.

Because scabies mimics several other itchy skin conditions, it often goes undiagnosed or misdiagnosed, particularly in nursing homes and extended care facilities where outbreaks may affect half or more of the patients. Various salves and lotions may alleviate your itching for a short period of time, but if scabies is the culprit, the mites will thrive, and often cause secondary infection requiring antibiotic therapy.

Once the proper diagnosis has been established—and only a physician is capable of recognizing it—the cure is relatively simple. Elimite Cream or Kwell (lindane) Lotion, prescription medications, will cure almost all cases of scabies with only one or two applications. (Do not use Kwell Lotion more than twice and do not use it on children under the age of six.) In addition, wash or dry clean all contaminated clothing and linens. And, since scabies spreads so swiftly, it is vitally important that every person in the household and all sex partners of the person affected should be treated whether or not they have any symptoms.

So if you have persistent, widespread itching that occurs below the neck, that is more pronounced at night, and that is unrelieved by the usual simple baths and lotions, see your dermatologist. Fortunately, the nasty scabies mite succumbs to a swift and simple cure.

For more information about lice and scabies, write to:
National Pediculosis Association
P.O. Box 149, Newton, MA 02161

800-446-4NPA; 617-449-6487
www.headlice.org or www.aad.org
or phone: 1-888-462-DERM x22

Recap

- Today lice have become a major public health problem throughout the world. Aggravated by poor living conditions, lack of personal cleanliness, and overcrowding, this infestation has reached epidemic proportions.
- Except for the common cold, head lice is the most frequently occurring communicable disease among children in the United States. Head lice have become especially prevalent in recent years, particularly among school children in urban areas.
- Scabies is a common and contagious skin disease. It has infested humans for at least 2,500 years. Like lice, it has reached epidemic proportions in the United States.

LICHEN PLANUS

Lichen planus is a relatively common, harmless, noncontagious, itchy rash that involves the skin and mucous membranes. Occurring most commonly in the middle years, it is characterized by reddish or violet-colored, firm, shiny, flat-topped, diamond-shaped "bumps" called papules.

The rash of lichen planus, occurring in about one percent of the population, is usually symmetrical in appearance and most often involves the inner surfaces of the wrists and forearms, the ankles, the genital areas, and the lower portion of the back. No area of the skin surface, however, is immune from this condition.

In the mouth, lichen planus can appear as a whitish or bluish-white, lacy-like pattern on the inner surface of the cheeks, or as whitish patches over the sides of the tongue. In rarer forms of this disorder, blisters or thickened warty areas may appear. In addition, one out of ten people with lichen planus have some type of nail changes, such as grooves, lines, distortion, or shedding of the nails.

The most characteristic symptom of lichen planus is itching. If there are only a few patches of the condition, the itching is usually mild. In the generalized form of the disease, however, the itching may become intense, causing loss of sleep, exhaustion, and despair.

The cause of lichen planus is unknown. It may be that it is not a disease at all—rather a symptom resulting from irritation, inflammation, or infection somewhere in the body.

Lichen planus can occur in people taking various drugs: high-blood pressure pills, antibiotics, and certain medications used to treat tuberculosis, malaria, and arthritis. The condition can also develop in workers in the photographic chemical industry following exposure to a type of color film developer. Many cases of resistant lichen planus occur in association with long-standing, untreated fungous infections of the feet (athlete's foot). Since the onset of lichen planus occasionally coincides with some major emotional upset, it is often thought to be triggered by prolonged worry, anxiety, fatigue, shock, or other stressful situation.

Lichen planus can last for years, but as a rule, the greater the involvement, the shorter the course. Generalized and extensive eruptions last anywhere from two months to two years or longer. Localized eruptions, on the other hand, have a tendency to remain considerably longer. Unfortunately, recurrences are common, so one is never sure that the condition has disappeared permanently.

While fairly common, lichen planus is not a condition that is easily recognized and diagnosed by the person who is afflicted. Or by relatives, friends, or the friendly pharmacist. Only a physician, specifically a dermatologist, can make an accurate diagnosis, and while there is no specific therapy for lichen planus, your physician will know how best to treat the rash and the itching that accompany it.

Available treatments include various cortisone-like creams applied locally, certain antihistamine-tranquilizers taken orally, and cortisone-like injections into the patches of lichen planus. None of these, however, has shown more than limited success.

If you have a rash that has been diagnosed by your physician as lichen planus, be content to know that it is not contagious, infectious, serious, or malignant. Get as much rest as possible and avoid worry, tension, and fatigue. Maintain your general health and correct any hidden, internal infection you may have, such as abscessed teeth or infected gums.

For further information about lichen planus, log on to
www.aad.org
1-888-462-DERM x22
or www.familydoctor.org/handouts/600.html

Recap

- The most characteristic symptom of lichen planus is itching. If there are only a few patches of the condition, the itching is usually mild.
- Lichen planus can last for years, but as a rule, the greater the involvement, the shorter the course. Generalized and extensive eruptions last anywhere from two months to two years or longer.
- Available treatments include various cortisone-like creams applied locally, certain antihistamine-tranquilizers taken orally, and cortisone-like injections into the patches of lichen planus.

LUPUS ERYTHEMATOSUS

"The wolf, I'm afraid, is inside tearing up the place. I've been in the hospital 50 days already this year."
—Flannery O'Connor, a few days before succumbing to her progressive fatal illness

Lupus erythematosus is one of those curious diseases that can masquerade as any of a dozen medical maladies. Its variety of symptoms include fever, chills, headache, weakness, fatigue, hair loss, joint pains, chest pains, epileptic seizures, personality changes, and rashes. Any or all of these symptoms may be part of this complicated disease we commonly call LE.

What exactly is LE? It is a chronic inflammation of connective tissue—the "body glue"—that binds our cells together. As such, it is considered a connective tissue, or collagen, disease. It's often classified in the rheumatic group of diseases along with rheumatic fever and rheumatoid arthritis. Every part of our bodies—organs, muscles, blood, joints, skin—has this connective tissue, and thus, may be affected by LE.

No one really knows what causes LE. This puzzling condition

131

affects over 500,000 people in the United States. It is most likely due to an "autoimmune process"—a technical way of saying that the body, due to some unexplained allergy, produces abnormal substances called autoantibodies, which attack and destroy its own tissues. Normally, when foreign substances (antigens), such as disease-producing germs or allergens, attack your body, it responds by producing antibodies to fight off these harmful invaders. In people with LE, this normal defense mechanism breaks down. And instead of attacking the antigens, the antibodies attack the body's own tissues.

It is important to know there are two types of LE. One is the benign or "friendly" type, called the discoid variety of LE. Triggered by some external factor, such as sunlight or injury, it shows up as red, scaly patches symmetrically distributed over the sun-exposed areas of the body—the cheeks, nose, ears, scalp, the backs of the hands, and occasionally the "V" of the neck. The patches of LE on the face thought to resemble the teeth marks of a wolf—hence the word lupus—can also affect the beard and scalp, usually resulting in permanent hair loss.

These patches grow larger over a period of months or years, forming disc-shaped (discoid) patches. They slowly lose their reddish color, and become white and depressed. This depression—essentially a scar—is the end result of a typical "discoid" lesion.

Discoid LE affects all races, is more common in young adults, and occurs twice as often in women as in men. If you have discoid LE, it's important to see a dermatologist. While the condition itself is relatively harmless, these "discs" may be harbingers of some underlying condition that can flare up into systemic lupus erythematosus (SLE).

SLE is a serious variety of LE that can affect and damage any or all of the body's organs or systems: kidneys, liver, heart, lungs, bone marrow, and joints. Fortunately, only about one in ten people with discoid LE ever progress to the systemic or internal type of the disease.

One of the triggering mechanisms that may convert the "friendly" condition into the more serious, "unfriendly" variety is sun exposure. People with LE, therefore, must strictly avoid the beaches, sunbathing in general, and tropical cruises.

Other factors that can turn the benign form of the disease into the more serious type are stress, injury, fatigue, overwork, certain medications such as those used for high blood pressure, heart disease, and epilepsy, antibiotics and birth control pills, various types of tranquilizers, and after exposure in tanning salons.

Treatment for LE will depend on your age and the nature and severity of your symptoms. Your dermatologist may prescribe cortisone-like creams and ointments to reduce the redness and relieve the inflammation in the affected patches. In rare cases, where the lesions are progressive, widespread, or disfiguring, your doctor may prescribe drugs called antimalarials, or other oral medications, to prevent further spread.

For further information regarding LE, contact:
National Lupus Erythematosus Foundation
2635 North First Street, Suite 206
San Jose, CA 95134
408-954-8600
or
The American Lupus Society
800-331-1802

Recap

- Lupus erythematosus is one of those curious diseases that can masquerade as any of a dozen other medical maladies.
- Discoid LE affects all races, is more common in young adults, and occurs twice as often in women as in men. If you have discoid LE, it's important to see a dermatologist.
- One of the triggering mechanisms that may convert the "friendly" condition into the more serious, "unfriendly" variety is sun exposure. People with LE, therefore, must strictly avoid the beaches, sunbathing in general, and tropical cruises.

RECTAL ITCH

"One bliss for which
There is no match
Is when you itch
To up and scratch."

133

Ogden Nash's little ditty doesn't include the socially unmentionable, embarrassing, persistent itch that torments the anal area, often incorrectly referred to as the rectal area. Known technically as pruritus ani (anal itch—itching of the anal region), this stubborn condition can cause sleepless nights, loss of work time, and severe emotional distress.

The single, most common cause of anal itch is poor anal hygiene. In most parts of Europe and in many Eastern countries this ailment is almost nonexistent. In these societies many people do not use toilet tissue—they *wash* the area. (The bidet is a much more distinctive sign of civilization than we would like to think!)

Other causes of anal itch include the following:

- Hemorrhoids (piles) and other rectal disease, such as fissures, fistulas, or discharge after rectal surgery.
- Chronic diarrhea.
- Fungal and yeast infections in the area—often associated with taking antibiotics over long periods.
- Pinworms and other parasitic infestations, such as lice (crabs) and mites (scabies).
- Psoriasis, seborrheic dermatitis, eczema.
- Warts in the anal area.
- Diabetes or liver disease.
- Certain foods, such as coffee, spicy foods, chocolate, raw fruits and vegetables, citrus fruits, and alcoholic beverages.
- Tight clothing—particularly the non-cotton varieties.
- Irritants that come into contact with the anal area, such as anesthetic ointments and suppositories used for piles; colored, perfumed, "moistened" and coarse toilet paper; soaps (especially the colored and scented varieties); deodorants; feminine hygiene sprays; bath salts; and—believe it or not—even nail polish has been implicated.
- Psychogenic causes. Anal itching occurs twice as often in men in their forties and fifties than in women of the same age. Physicians believe this to be a result of certain stress situations (monetary for the most part) that develop in middle-aged men.

And then there are those cases where one cannot determine the cause—where painstaking study has failed to reveal any causative factor. This is by far the most common situation, and, as a result, the most resistant to treatment.

If you have prolonged, continuous, intolerable anal itching, see your family physician. For temporary relief, here are a few things you can do:

- Never use dry toilet paper. Instead, use cotton balls soaked in warm water. And never wipe or rub! Blotting or patting is enough. And make sure the area is kept scrupulously dry.
- Never use soap while you have "the itch." Use a mild cleanser such as Cetaphil Cleanser.
- Avoid irritating substances, such as bath salts, deodorants, sprays, and perfumes. And do not dry your clothes with those fabric softener sheets.
- Avoid tight, underwear, pajamas, and pants. Wear only loose, cotton clothes on your bottom half. Boxer shorts; not jockey shorts for men.
- If you suspect that diet may be responsible for your itch, cut out spicy foods, chocolate, coffee, alcohol, popcorn, and raw fruit and vegetables.
- Avoid antibiotics, laxatives, and mineral oil.
- Don't apply any over-the-counter salves and suppositories to the anal area, especially those containing benzocaine and other -caine derivatives. These may only aggravate your malady.
- If you find that you itch more at night, wear a pair of soft cotton gloves when you retire.
- If you suspect that emotional stress and tension are the cause, simmer down, stay cool, and relax.

For the severe, acute anal itch, your physician will probably prescribe baths in hot water, a special prescription cream or ointment, and perhaps an anti-itch pill to break that itch-scratch reflex.

How can you prevent anal itching? No problem. Keep the area scrupulously clean at all times and wash with a mild soap and water, or a gentle cleanser, at least once daily (particularly after a bowel movement). Dry the area with soft, white toilet tissue. (Rabelais wrote that wiping the anal skin with the neck of a plump, downy, warm goose was unquestionably "the most lordly, excellent, and expedient technique ever seen." Soft toilet paper is considerably easier to use, much cheaper, and probably works as well!)

If you follow the cleansing and drying method just described, you may never again have to "up and scratch."

For further information about rectal itch, log on to www.aad.org
1-888-462-DERM x22

Recap

- The single, most common cause of anal itch is poor anal hygiene.
- Anal itching occurs twice as often in men in their 40s and 50s than in women of the same age. Physicians believe this to be a result of certain stress situations that develop in middle-aged men.
- Don't apply any over-the-counter salves and suppositories to the anal area, especially those containing benzocaine and other -caine derivatives. These may only aggravate your malady.

ROSACEA

Rosacea is a chronic skin disorder, affecting more than 14 million people in the United States, that is distinguished by flushing of the face, by acne-like pimples and pustules, and by small thin veins that course over the skin of the cheeks and nose. It can be most embarrassing to those who suffer from this disorder, as it is frequently associated with alcohol consumption.

It is typically a problem of middle-aged women around the time of menopause, but when men blossom forth with rosacea, cosmetically disagreeable complications can arise (see below). Light complexion and blue eyes seem to predispose to rosacea. Many of those affected come from the Celtic regions—Ireland, Scotland, England, as well as northern Germany.

Many well-known people have been and are afflicted with rosacea: the late Princess Diana, President Clinton, Rembrandt, J.P. Morgan and, of course, W.C. Fields, the one with the bulbous nose attributed to his constant drinking.

The rash of rosacea, resembling the acne pimples of teenagers, is usually symmetrically distributed over the forehead, cheeks, nose, chin, rims of ears, and can involve the eyelids.

Beginning as a flushing or a stinging, it gradually evolves into pimples, knobby lumps on the nose (in men), and thin red lines over the nose and cheeks as a result of enlarged blood vessels.

The cause of rosacea is an enigma, but we do know that various stimuli—hot and spicy foods, alcoholic beverages, coffee, increased environmental temperature, and even emotional tension—can lead to a dilatation, a widening, of the blood vessels of the face, resulting in exaggeration of the normal flush response. This repeated flushing and blushing is followed by permanent redness. In advanced cases, unsightly pimples, pustules, and fine veins will materialize.

Certain medications are also known to bring about rosacea: ACE-Inhibitors, Vasotec, Capoten, Prinivil, Zestril, Accupril, Altase, niacin and others.

Rosacea is occasionally associated with gastrointestinal disturbances. Often there is thought to be a small mite (Demodex folliculorum) that thrives and multiplies in the oil glands of the skin, which seems to be implicated in many of these pustular infections. In long-standing, severe cases, a cosmetic disfigurement of the nose—rhinophyma—can develop. This condition is especially pronounced in elderly males. The nose becomes enlarged, the tissue becomes soft, and the openings of the oil glands become widened and plugged with a cheese-like material.

Rosacea-like inflammation can be a result of using strong cortisone-like topical creams and lotions on the facial skin for extended periods of time. At one time Helicobacter pylori was thought to play a role in roscoe, but this has been effectively disproved.

Rosacea treatment aims at eliminating all stimuli—the so-called "tripwires"—that encourage the widening of the superficial blood vessels of the face:

- No alcoholic beverages, especially red wine, gin, vodka, beer and bourbon.
- No spicy foods.
- No liver, dairy products, tomatoes or any other food that you think will cause an aggravation of the condition.

- No very hot foods or drinks.
- No coffee.
- No exposure to heat or cold.
- Avoid the sun like the plague!
- Steer clear of saunas, hot baths, exercise.
- Various skin care products: fragrances, perfumes, hair sprays, topical cortisone preparations can also exacerbate rosacea.

While there is no cure for rosacea, it can be controlled. Dermatologists usually treat rosacea with oral antibiotics, such as tetracycline, doxycycline, minocycline or erythromycin, as well as with various types of surface remedies containing metronidazole. Some of the topical preparations containing metronidazole are MetroGel, MetroCream, and MetroLotion, all prescription products. Applied twice daily—even without oral antibiotics—a marked improvement can be expected from these topical medications in a matter of a few weeks for all degrees of rosacea.

When exposed to the sun, always use a sunscreen with an SPF of at least 15 (see Chapter on Sun).

If left untreated, rosacea may gradually increase in severity, infect the eyelids and eyes—ocular rosacea—and can last for years.

For further information concerning rosacea write to or phone:
The National Rosacea Society
800 South Northwest Highway, Suite 200
Barrington, IL 60010
1-800-NO-BLUSH
www.rosacea.org or www.aad.org
1-888-462-DERM x22

Recap

- Rosacea is a chronic skin disorder affecting more than 14 million people in the United States, which is distinguished by a flushed face, acne-like pimples and pustules, and by small thin veins that course over the skin of the cheeks and nose.
- Rosacea is typically a problem of middle-aged women around the time of menopause.

- The treatment of rosacea aims at eliminating all stimuli—the so-called "tripwires"—that encourage the widening of the superficial blood vessels of the face.

SEBORRHEIC DERMATITIS

Seborrheic dermatitis is a fancy name for what I refer to as "dandruff of the skin."

Characterized by symmetrically distributed, red, scaly, and greasy patches seborrheic dermatitis is a condition—not really a disease—that dermatologists can diagnose just by looking at you. It doesn't take fancy blood tests, sophisticated laboratory analyses, or microscopic examination to prove conclusively that you have seborrheic dermatitis. All it takes is a dermatologist's scrupulous eye. Seborrheic dermatitis, affecting between 3 percent and 5 percent of the population, is one of the most common skin disorders seen by practicing dermatologists. It affects people with Parkinson's disease and about 90 percent of those infected with HIV (human immunodeficiency virus). It is not serious, infectious, contagious or malignant.

As with hundreds of skin ailments, no one knows what causes this mainly cosmetic problem. There are many theories, including the following:

- a hormonal imbalance.
- a hereditary predisposition.
- dietary indiscretions and obesity.
- drugs (Thorazine, Haldol, Tagamet, anti-seizure medications).
- environmental factors.
- germs.
- emotional stress and tension, worry, loss of sleep.
- certain nervous disorders.
- a yeast-like organism related to a fungus.

A recent theory proposes that seborrheic dermatitis results from a defect in your body's defense against certain germs that live on the surface of your skin. Actually, no one knows…

There is a condition in infants called "cradle cap," where the scalp is covered with thick, yellowish-brown, greasy crusts. The hair becomes sticky and matted. This common disorder is thought to be due to leftover hormones that have been passed on to the susceptible infant from his or her mother. These maternal hormones stimulate the sebaceous (oil) glands in the scalp, with the result that there is a marked production of an oily secretion—sebum. This sebum is responsible for "cradle cap"—the earliest manifestation of seborrheic dermatitis.

Shortly after birth, activity in these sebaceous glands diminishes. The result is that you will almost never have seborrheic dermatitis during your childhood. When you reach puberty, however, your developing sex glands begin to stimulate these quiescent "oil formers," which then increase in size and become very active. If you have seborrheic dermatitis, you will notice that the condition begins on your scalp in the form of redness and diffuse scaling.

In addition to this "heavy dandruff" the hair gets greasy, and the scalp may itch. Scaly, pink, crust-like patches may begin to form around your hairline. Other areas of your body rich in oil glands often develop patches as well: your eyebrows, the areas over and behind your ears, your ear canals, the sides of your nose, your forehead, your chest and armpits.

If you are a young man, you may develop these patches in your beard, your sideburns, and your mustache area. In certain cases, you may have the rash on your chest, back, and pubic region. Some people develop it in the body folds: the groins, the armpits, under the breasts, and in the bellybutton.

Your rash may or may not itch.

A special case of seborrheic dermatitis occurs when the margins of the eyelids become red and covered with small white scales or yellowish crusts.

Since seborrheic dermatitis is a chronic and recurring condition, flare-ups at odd moments are common. These occur more often in colder months.

Treatment of seborrheic dermatitis is directed at minimizing the symptoms, rather than curing the disorder permanently. Persistent, regular treatment should control this annoying ailment.

Here are a dozen suggestions for managing and living with your seborrheic dermatitis:

- Shampoo frequently—daily if at all possible. Frequent shampooing is the first rule in treating seborrheic dermatitis. Some of the over-the-counter shampoos that dermatologists recommend are those with tar, zinc, selenium sulfide, ketoconazole, or salicylic acid.
- Since the patches of seborrheic dermatitis are prone to secondary infection by bacteria and other germs, keep your skin clean by washing carefully and regularly using a mild cleanser such as Cetaphil Cleanser.
- Keep "cool." Avoid stress and emotional tension.
- Get plenty of rest.
- Eat a well-balanced diet.
- Avoid greasy foods and alcoholic beverages.
- If you are overweight, try to lose those extra pounds.
- Avoid greasy cosmetics and oily moisturizers.
- If it itches, try not to scratch.
- Exposure to small amounts of sunlight usually helps, but since the sun's rays have potential serious side effects, do so in moderation.
- If you are under the care of a dermatologist, follow his or her instructions for the proper use of topical medications.
- Avoid over-the-counter remedies that have not been recommended by your doctor.

Specific treatment for seborrheic dermatitis will depend on the location and degree of the rash. In mild cases of seborrheic dermatitis, when the scalp alone is affected, conscientious shampooing with an anti-dandruff shampoo may be enough. In stubborn cases and when patches are extensive, you should consult your dermatologist.

The time-honored topical medications used in treating seborrheic dermatitis are sulfur, tar, salicylic acid, and low-strength cortisone-type creams. Many of these must be prescribed by your dermatologist. Some dermatologists, believing a fungus causes the condition, will prescribe Nizoral, an antifungal cream.

For the stubborn variety of this common ailment, other methods—injections, stronger cortisone-like creams and lotions, and other topical preparations—may be necessary.

For more information about seborrheic dermatitis, contact:
National Institute of Arthritis & Musculoskeletal & Skin Diseases
National Institutes of Health
1 AMS Circle
Bethesda, MD 20892-3675
301-495-4484
www.nih.gov/niams or www.aad.org
or www.familydoctor.org/handouts/157.html
1-888-462-DERM x22

Recap

- Seborrheic dermatitis affects between 3 percent to 5 percent of the population. It is one of the most common skin disorders seen by practicing dermatologists. "Cradle cap" is the earliest manifestation of seborrheic dermatitis.
- A special case of seborrheic dermatitis occurs when the margins of the eyelids become red and covered with small white scales or yellowish crusts.
- In mild cases of seborrheic dermatitis, when the scalp is the only area affected, frequent and conscientious shampooing with an anti-dandruff shampoo may be all you need.

5 Hair and Hair Care

HAIR AND HAIR CARE

Hair—our crowning glory.

And yet, depending on where it grows, how much, and upon whom, hair can be a blessing or a curse.

We cut it, shave it, twirl it, comb it, and brush it to make it appear longer and more abundant. Some tease, tint, dye, bleach, spray, iron, roll, and frost it. We straighten curly hair, and we curl straight hair. Brunettes become blonds, and vice versa.

We tear our hair. We split hairs. We let our hair down. We make our hair stand on end, and we get into someone else's hair.

What is this culturally, socially, and sexually significant ornamental appendage we refer to as hair? It is a nonliving, protein fiber—a strong, elastic thread, arising from a long indentation—a follicle, or "pore"—in the skin.

Hair is dead. Although it is as integral a component of the body as our skin, once it has emerged from the follicle, it is no longer nourished by a blood supply or by any other life-giving bodily fluids.

What, then, is its purpose? Thousands of years ago our forebears were covered with hair in much the same manner as the monkeys and apes. It was a protective barrier against the elements: sun, wind, extremes of heat and cold, rain, snow, and insects. It also acted as a cushion to protect against the force of bumps, abrasions, and blows in battle.

143

As we evolved, our need for hair gradually diminished. We developed clothing, which protected us from the ravages of nature, and body hair became redundant. Today, except for eyebrows and eyelashes, which act as a sieve against insects, dust, and irritants, hair serves no biological function. It is not essential to physical health.

Hair varies in color, texture, length, and type among different races. It is second only to skin as a physical sign of racial difference. Asians, Eskimos, and Native Americans have sparse facial and body hair, and straight, dark hairs on their heads. African blacks have slightly more body hair and woolly or wiry hair on their scalps. American blacks, who are often mixtures of other races, have straight, wavy, curly, fine, or coarse hair on their heads. Whites have more body hair than any other race and have curly, wavy, or straight, fine hair on their heads.

As a rule, we each have three types of hair: the long, soft, terminal hairs, such as those on the scalp, armpits, and pubic region; the short, stiff, coarse hairs of the eyelids, eyebrows, nose, and ears; and the soft, fine, downy fuzz (known as lanugo or vellus hairs) which covers much of the rest of our bodies. Our only "hairless" regions are the palms and soles, the lips, the nipples, and certain parts of the genitals.

All of us are born with a fixed number of hair follicles that remain with us—on our heads, in our armpits, on our faces and bodies—for an entire lifetime. There are about five million hair follicles found throughout the human body. Each hair follicle is supplied by one or more oil glands that produce a secretion that gives your hair its richness and gloss. The number of hair follicles—and therefore, hairs—is inherited. In other words, if your parents had 100,000 hairs on their heads, the chances are that you will have approximately the same number.

Blonds may or may not have more fun than everyone else, but they do have more hair. They average about 120,000 scalp hairs, while brunettes have about 100,000, and redheads only 80,000. To compensate for this disparity, blond hairs are fine and red hairs are thick. If we weighed the total number of scalp hairs from an average blond, they would weigh roughly the same as those of a redhead! Although fine hair is a nuisance and a bother, blonds, since they have more hair on their heads, can afford to lose more; and, because there's more of it, fine hair has a tendency to go gray more slowly.

About 90 percent of a person's scalp hair is continually growing. Ten percent of the scalp hair is in a resting stage that lasts about two months. At the end of this resting phase, the hair is shed. Hair loss on the scalp in normal, healthy people varies from about 50 to 120 strands daily. In other words, in the course of a year you'll lose about 30,000 hairs from your scalp. All of these hairs are constantly being replaced, at least until the aging process occurs, and certain hormonal changes begin to occur.

Most scalp hairs grow about one-half inch per month, so it takes about two years to grow shoulder-length hair. Each strand, however, does not grow indefinitely. If you never had your hair cut, it would only grow about two-and-one-half feet. After a period of time, usually two to four years, the hair follicle that produces the individual hair gets tired and stops working. The strand stops growing and eventually falls out, to be replaced by a new "working" hair when the follicle has renewed itself.

Hair grows faster in warm weather, slows down during illness or pregnancy, and falls out more in autumn when "the leaves on the trees begin to drop," as it were. Contrary to popular myths and superstitions, hair does not grow thicker or faster when cut or shaved. Nor does it grow after death. In one year, the body produces seven miles of hair—350 miles in an average lifetime.

The following sections cover some basics that can help you have healthier looking hair as well as cope with some common conditions that affect our scalp and hair, such as dandruff, seborrheic dermatitis, too little hair, and too much hair.

HAIR CARE

Compare your hair to a cashmere sweater. How long would that sweater last if you constantly washed, shampooed, combed, brushed, colored, tinted, bleached, teased, straightened, curled, rolled, pulled, twisted, and twirled it? What if you consistently exposed it to the sun, wind, rain, snow, sleet and extremes of heat and cold? How about if you wore it swimming in polluted lakes and streams and chlorinated pools, and then got it steamed, ironed, sprayed, flipped, oiled, wound, feathered, swirled, dipped, stripped, frosted, perfumed, frizzed, fuzzed, matted, braided, and waxed. And *then* blown dry by

1500 watts of hot air? How long would it last? A month? A week?

Your hair goes through this and more. Yet, barring certain diseases and conditions, it lasts a lifetime.

Taking good care of your hair, however, can make a big difference in how it looks during its "lifetime." Healthy looking, attractive hair requires consistent, responsible care and conditioning, good diet, and exercise. It also requires keeping stress and emotional tensions to a minimum. (Remember, I did not say *healthy* hair; I said *healthy looking* hair. How can something that's dead be healthy?)

Many young women and men consult a dermatologist because they're concerned about a change in the growth or appearance of their hair. More often than not, the change is the result of abuse, rather than disease.

What causes breakage of hair? Often, it is related to physical damage. Here are some factors that can physically "injure" your hair:

- Brushes with sharp bristles.
- Metal or plastic combs.
- Braiding your hair tightly.
- Winding your hair tightly.
- Using brush rollers.
- Backcombing.
- Repeated wetting and blow-drying.
- Repeated manipulation.
- Wearing tight hats, caps, and headbands.
- Excessive sun exposure, which "weathers" the hair by injuring its keratin (protein) fibers.

Chemical injury is probably the most common cause of hair breakage. When the outer keratin layer of the hair shaft (the cuticle) is exposed to chemical attack—from bleaches, hair straighteners, permanent hair dyes, thioglycolate wave solutions, etc.—it develops a stiff, straw-like texture, making it more susceptible to breakage.

To prevent breakage and maintain a healthier-looking head of hair, avoid as much physical injury to the hair shaft as possible. Hair "wears out" anyway, and increased manipulation, in any form, speeds up the process. Here are some specific tips:

- Brush and comb less often. ("One-hundred-strokes-a-day"

brushing or combing is *not* good for your hair.)
- Don't backcomb .
- No braids or ponytails.
- Use pure bristle brushes and hard rubber combs.
- Don't wear tight hats, caps, or headbands.
- Use a mild, gentle shampoo.
- Use crème rinses or conditioners.
- Trim split and damaged ends.

A word about shampooing:

Good hair care begins with shampooing. The frequency of shampooing is an individual affair. You may shampoo daily or oftener, if need be, without harming the hair or hair follicle in any way.

If your hair is oily, or if you live in the city where you are constantly exposed to inordinate amounts of dust, grease, grime, soot, and other chemical pollutants, you should shampoo often, with a good commercial shampoo—not with bar soap.

An important and little known fact about shampooing is that to derive benefit from it the shampoo should be massaged into the entire scalp for *at least* five minutes—preferably longer—using fairly hot water. Thorough rinsing is a must. For those who like a crème rinse, I recommend using it in moderation; small amounts prevent the "greasies."

If you blowdry your hair, follow the manufacturer's directions and make sure to keep the blow dryer at least six inches away from your head.

MYTHS & MISCONCEPTIONS PERTAINING TO THE HAIR

- *If you cut, pluck, or shave your hair, it will grow back longer and thicker and faster.*
  Hair is a dead protein thread. Once it emerges from the hair follicle, it has no blood supply, no life, and cannot be changed!

- *"Eat your crusts of bread. They will make your hair curly."*
  No way!

- *"Rub a new penny over the ends of your **hair**, and your **hair** will quickly grow long."*
  Answer: No way!

147

- *If you cut your **hair** in "the waxing of the moon," your **hair** will have a fine texture.*
  Answer: No way!

- *"If your **hair** is tangled, rats have slept in it."*
  Answer: What do you think?

- *To prevent baldness, wash your **hair** with wild grapevine blossom tea.*
  Answer: No way!

- Finally, the so-called "hair analysis" is an unreliable method of diagnosing nutritional problems and exposure to environmental toxins. Don't get sucked into having your hair "analyzed."

Recap

- Hair is a dead protein thread. Although it is as integral a component of the body as our skin, once it has emerged from the follicle, it is no longer nourished by a blood supply or by any other life-giving bodily fluids.
- All of us are born with a fixed number of hair follicles that remain with us—on our heads, in our armpits, on our faces and bodies—for an entire lifetime.
- Contrary to popular myths and superstitions, hair does not grow thicker or faster or longer when cut or shaved. Nor does it grow after death.

DANDRUFF

"Nothing stops dandruff like a blue serge suit."

Blue serge may be a little before your time, but the saying still has more than a speck of truth to it.

Dandruff is a normal condition. Everyone has it to some degree. It's only when the scaling or flaking of dandruff shows up like stardust on the collar of that dark suit or dress that you may become embarrassed and concerned.

To understand dandruff, you have to know a little about the epidermis, the upper layer of the skin. Like all cells in the body, skin cells are manufactured constantly to replace those that have outlived their usefulness and died. In normal skin, the process for a cell to be born, move to the outer edge of the skin surface, and then flake off takes about a month. Subsequent flake-off takes about a month. Dead cells are being continually sloughed off as new ones are being pushed up from the deeper layers in a neverending process of cell division. This cycle, at a faster rate, gives rise to the tiny scaly flakes you continuously shed from the entire skin surface.

You can control this normal periodic scaling on the scalp by frequent shampooing with any commercial shampoo. In the abnormal process, however, the cells are born and die at a much faster rate, resulting in flaking and sometimes even redness and itching. To control this moderately severe type of dandruff will probably require something other than the usual over-the-counter anti-dandruff remedies.

No one really knows what causes flaking to get out of control. Many theories have been proposed: hormone imbalance, germs (bacteria and fungi) living on the scalp, excessive production of oil from the oil glands, dietary indiscretions and deficiencies, allergies, poor hygiene, irritation and inflammation from cosmetics and chemicals, hereditary influences, and emotional stress. One rarely sees dandruff in children under the age of twelve, which leads us to suspect that some type of hormone influences the condition. There is no clear-cut proof, however, to support any of these theories.

We do know, however, that dandruff is not contagious (you can't pick it up from someone's comb), it does not lead to any serious scalp problem, and it does NOT cause baldness.

There are dozens of shampoos available for the relief of simple dandruff. But remember, you never really get "rid" of it, since your scalp makes a new supply of flakes approximately every three days.

No one shampoo is good for everybody. Where you live, the type of water in your home, your particular kind of hair—all play a role in the effectiveness of a shampoo.

Medicated shampoos usually contain sulfur, zinc, ketoconazole, salicylic acid, selenium, tar, or some combination thereof. Your pharmacist can offer you a variety of these preparations. Find the one you feel is most effective, and stick with it.

If your dandruff is persistent and doesn't respond to conscientious shampooing, check with your dermatologist. You may have seborrheic dermatitis, psoriasis or some other condition that requires medical attention.

For further information about dandruff, log on to www.aad.org
1-888-462-DERM x22

Recap

- Dandruff is a normal condition. Everyone has it to some degree.
- Dandruff is not contagious, you can't pick it up from someone's comb, it does not lead to any serious scalp problem, and it does NOT cause baldness.
- If your dandruff is persistent and doesn't respond to frequent shampooing, check with your dermatologist. You may have seborrheic dermatitis, psoriasis, or some other condition that requires medical expertise.

HAIR LOSS AND EXCESS HAIR

A certain amount of hair loss is an inevitable part of the aging process in most everybody. Since it is asymptomatic, leaves no visible scarring, and results in no physiologic functions of the individual, it is really not a disease. Shall we call it a disorder? Or is it, in the words of James Joyce, "the ineluctable modality of the visible?" Hair loss happens!

Some studies have suggested that varying degrees of hair loss— too much hair in unwanted areas; loss or thinning of scalp hair—are associated with negative effects on quality of life in some people.

In the following chapters we will touch on some of the problems of hair loss and excess hair in both women and men.

FEMALE HAIR LOSS

Are young American women having a collective "bad hair day?" Are American women becoming *bald?*

There is no clear-cut answer to this pressing problem. We do know, however, that in the past few decades there has been an increase in complaints from young women about hair loss—steady, progressive, diffuse, mysterious hair loss. This female pattern hair loss is quite common, beginning in the late twenties, reaching almost 30 percent in women over thirty years of age. There are very few medical conditions that produce more emotional trauma than thinning of scalp hair in healthy young and middle-aged women.

Years ago, doctors rarely saw cases of female hair loss. But recently, young women have begun to notice an increase in the number of hairs lost with each grooming—on the comb, in the brush, in the washbasin. After months or years, there is visible thinning—a euphemism for baldness.

The healthy scalp loses between 50 and 120 hairs daily. This loss, let me reassure you, is balanced by continuous regrowth. When the rate of hair loss, however, exceeds the rate of new growth, thinning and balding become apparent.

As a rule, it is not excessive hair loss, rather an underproduction of new hair that results in thinning. The lack of production of new, viable hair can be traced to several different sources.

Major factors in female pattern hair loss are hormonal changes, heredity, and the aging process. Hormonal changes are those that occur after childbirth, and with certain types of endocrine tumors and imbalances (thyroid trouble, ovarian problems, and other hormone conditions). In addition, if you are taking the low-dose birth control pill, you may be experiencing hair loss.

Hereditary factors also play a strong role in pattern hair loss. If your mother or grandmother had sparse hair, it is likely that you (and possibly your daughter) may suffer from the same deficiency.

Finally, the aging process (due to diminished production of female hormones) is a strong factor in female hair loss. After producing for so many decades, the hair follicles become weak, tired, and sluggish. Some of them fade away and produce no more—one of the prices we must pay for growing old.

Recent thinning and balding in women is due to environmental changes and the products used for beautification. Here are some examples:

- Mechanical tension and violence on the hair shaft due to new hairstyles and cosmetic aids. These cause injury to the hair follicle and, when prolonged, interfere with the scalp's circulation.

- Excessive chemical exposure associated with hair styling (for example, cold-wave solutions, bleaches, and hair straightening products), and increased exposure to synthetic detergents and additives in commercial shampoos, dyes, and hair sprays.
- Nutritional deficiencies in "crash-dieters," in vegetarians who suffer protein malnutrition, and in those suffering from iron-deficiency anemia.
- General anesthesia during surgical operations.
- Various drugs used to treat cancer, and anticoagulants (blood thinners) used in heart disease. Other drugs that may cause hair loss are ACE-inhibitors, beta-blocking agents, cholesterol-lowering drugs (Pravachol, Zocor, Lipitor), antidepressants, high doses of vitamin A, and dozens of others. If you have any doubts about whether or not a medication can cause hair loss, ask your physician or pharmacist.
- Emotional stress and tension are believed to impair the circulation of the hair follicle.

What's a woman to do? Here are a few basic rules for healthy hair:

- Shampoo your hair regularly, daily if at all possible.
- Use only pure bristle brushes and hard rubber combs. Don't use the plastic or metal varieties.
- Reduce mechanical manipulation of the hair shaft; avoid teasing and ratting, vigorous combing and brushing; tight, restrictive hairstyles; tight braids and ponytails; and excessive hot combing. Hair responds best to gentle care.
- Avoid excessive bleaching, dyeing, and straightening.
- Keep up your general health, avoid crash diets, and cut down on smoking.
- If you are taking the low-dose birth control pill, ask your gynecologist if you may change these to the higher-dose variety.
- Avoid emotional stress and tension.

There is a topical medication—Rogaine for Women—that purportedly stops excess hair loss and promotes hair growth. It is an over-the-counter medication but if you use it, you must use it forever. Check with your dermatologist anyway, if you are interested. He or she may be able to give you more information regarding this topical preparation.

Other than Rogaine, don't be misled by advertisements and commercials for potions and unguents that promise to grow hair. They do not work.

I also advocate taking a multivitamin-mineral supplement along with Biotin Forte 3 milligrams—nothing less than 3 milligrams will work!—on a daily basis.

Finally, if your situation does not improve, see your dermatologist. There may be some infection, hormonal imbalance, or medication responsible.

And remember: women don't get bald the way men do. While you may have to get used to a thinner crop when you are in your forties, it is highly unlikely you will lose all of your "crowning glory."

For further information about hair loss, log on to www.aad.org
or www.familydoctor.org/handouts/061.html
1-888-462-DERM x22

Recap

- In the past few decades there has been a mysterious increase in complaints at dermatologists' offices, from young women with progressive, diffuse hair loss.
- The healthy scalp loses between 50 and 120 hairs daily. The loss is balanced out by continuous regrowth. However, when the rate of hair loss exceeds the rate of new growth, thinning and balding become apparent.
- Heredity plays a strong role in pattern hair loss. If your mother or grandmother had sparse hair, it is likely that you (and possibly your daughter) may suffer from the same deficiency.

MALE BALDNESS

"Ugly are hornless bulls, a field without grass is an eyesore,
So is a tree without leaves, so is a head without hair."
—Ovid, *The Art of Love*

Male baldness may be a joke on TV, in the movies, and at parties, but for many young men who mourn every lost strand, facing the prospect of premature baldness is no joke at all. It can be a source of great anxiety, a personal loss, and a profoundly depressing experience, which diminishes one's self-image. To some, the fountain of youth is no more than a head full of dead protein threads.

Would it comfort you to know that Caesar was bald? Did Yul Brynner and Kojak look unhappy?

The hirsute male has always been a symbol of virility and physical strength. The biblical Samson, the Greek Hercules, Zeus, and Poseidon were men and gods of prodigious strength, represented as powerful, hairy, and bearded—but so are gorillas!

Male pattern baldness, one of man's greatest fears, affects well over half the adult male population in America and is so common that we consider some degree of hair loss in adult males normal. Would it console you to know that hair loss has absolutely no adverse effect on virility? Or on potency? Or on strength? Would it help you to know there are some disadvantages to long hair? It can obstruct your vision. It collects dandruff and, occasionally, small creatures such as lice! The only harmful effect of premature hair loss is psychological. It may encourage loss of confidence and, with it, anxiety, stress, and depression.

The cause and extent of male baldness, while not completely understood, depends on three factors: inheritance, age, and male hormones. If your parents and/or grandparents had this bald trait, the chances are that you will inherit it. Once begun, it is a progressive condition; the older you get, the more hair you will lose.

You'll be surprised to know that when you get bald, you actually don't lose any of your hair. In fact, you go to the grave with the same number of hair follicles with which you were born! What the balding man loses are the longer, darker, coarser hairs that have been replaced with soft, downy fuzz, called vellus hairs.

Medical science so far has been helpless in reversing, arresting, or curing this pattern. There is, however, a great deal of research about fattening and lengthening those downy, vellus hairs. A recent study has found that a protein—vascular endothelial growth factor (VEGF)—helps the body grow blood vessels. And since blood circulation is associated with hair growth, it may be that this new experimental drug made into a cream, lotion or ointment will help men grow longer and thicker hairs, replacing the small, downy peach fuzz. It's working in mice; it might work in humans. We are working on it…

And, lest you be sadly misled, there are no salves, lotions, shampoos, vitamins, or natural food supplements that will grow hair where there are no hair follicles. Hair "restorers" are for the birds—not for the scalp.

Years ago, it was demonstrated that the female hormone estrogen, when rubbed into the scalp, could lengthen the peach fuzz appreciably and slow down or reduce the rate of pattern baldness. But men should think twice about the side effects of estrogen. Do you want larger breasts? A high-pitched voice? A diminished sexual appetite? How would more hair look with these acccessories?

There are, however, two drugs that have shown some limited promise. One, minoxidil, has been used orally for people who are afflicted with severe high blood pressure. How minoxidil—the brand name is Rogaine—helps high blood pressure or how it helps grow hair is not precisely known. It probably acts as a vasodilator, a chemical that expands blood vessels, by bringing nourishing blood to normally deprived hair follicle cells.

Among oral minoxidil's many undesirable side effects is hypertrichosis—the growth of excess hair—that is noted in about 80 percent of the patients taking the drug. Dermatologists have "tamed" this powerful chemical and fashioned it into a lotion, which grows hair when rubbed into bald spots.

The latest reports show that young men under the age of 26 who are using this product—Rogaine—do much better than older men. It rarely works at all for a receding hairline; it can best restore hair on the crown of the head but not at the temples. The hairs—if any—that do grow are little more than wispy strands, no one in the studies developed a full head of hair.

If you are interested, ask your dermatologist about it. It is a nonprescription medication, is relatively expensive, and must be used forever. When it is discontinued, any hair that had begun to grow will fall out within three or four months. Its very rare adverse side effects include fainting, vomiting, rapid heartbeat, and difficulty breathing.

Another newly approved drug is finasteride. This oral medication, the trade name is Propecia, is purported to grow hair successfully in balding men. The side effects of finasteride are minimal, but if a man embarks on this method of treatment, it must be kept up forever. (Finasteride—under the name Proscar—is also used in men who suffer from enlarged prostate glands.)

So what does that leave for the despondent young man? A hair transplant? A wig? Or the confidence in knowing that bald may be beautiful; that the high brow, the egghead and the chrome dome, marks of internal wisdom, are "in."

For further information about hair loss, log on to www.aad.org or www.familydoctor.org/handouts/061.html
1-888-462-DERM x22

Recap

- Male pattern baldness, which continues to be one of man's greatest fears, affects well over half the adult male population in America and is so common that we consider some degree of hair loss in adult males normal.
- The cause and extent of male baldness, while not completely understood, depends on three factors: inheritance, age, and male hormones. If your parents and/or grandparents had this bald trait, chances are that you will inherit it.
- Be confident in knowing that bald may be beautiful and that the high brow, the egghead and the "chrome dome"—the marks of internal wisdom—are "in."

ALOPECIA AREATA

Bogie noticed a bare spot on his cheek where his beard was not growing. The one spot increased to several—then he'd wake in the morning and find clumps of hair on the pillow....A visit to the doctor was in order. The verdict was that he had a disease known as alopecia areata—in layman's terms, hair falls out....His next film was going to be *The Treasure of the Sierra Madre* with John Huston, and he'd have to wear a wig....

—From *"Lauren Bacall, By Myself"*

It goes by the lilting name alopecia areata, but patchy hair loss, as it's commonly called, would not be desirable by any name. Still, it can be treated, so don't despair.

Patchy hair loss is pretty much what it says it is—a condition of the scalp and other hairy areas of the body that begins with the sudden appearance of one or more small, round or oval bald patches, which gradually enlarge over a period of weeks. It affects all age groups but is more common among children and young adults.

The bald patches appear rather quickly on an otherwise healthy, hairy area. They do not itch, burn, or cause any pain. The scalp is the most commonly affected area, but alopecia areata can affect the beard, eyebrows, eyelashes, and any other hairy region. The hairs at the periphery of these balding patches are usually loose and easily pulled out.

In severe cases, patches on the scalp become so large that they merge to produce a total loss of the scalp hair. This is alopecia totalis. In rare cases, the condition may progress until every hair over the entire body falls out—alopecia universalis. Queen Elizabeth I of England contracted this condition in 1562 following her severe bout with smallpox. She was completely bald for the remainder of her life and resorted to wigs and other artifices.

No one knows why the hair root on some people simply stops making hair. I explain to my patients that while the hair growing "equipment" is in no way damaged, the "hair-growth switch" has been turned off. And once the switch has been turned back on, renewed hair growth will take place.

Theories have linked alopecia areata to certain hormonal changes, blows to the head, and severe emotional strain or shock. In some cases it runs in families. The latest theory is that alopecia areata may be an autoimmune disorder, a type of "self-allergy," where the body rejects its own tissue, in this case, the hair follicle.

Fortunately, for many people, alopecia areata is a temporary, self-limiting affliction. Even without treatment, the hairs often begin to grow back slowly after a few weeks or months. At first, the regrowth occurs as fine, downy white hairs. Eventually these hairs develop their normal texture and color. The course is erratic and unpredictable. As a rule, however, the greater the initial hair loss and the earlier in life it begins, the more likely it is to persist or recur.

Is there any treatment for alopecia areata, and can we turn the "switch" back on? Yes.

First of all, stop worrying. Make sure that your general health is good. Only your physician can correct any deficiencies and give you a "clean bill of health."

Other treatments include injections of certain cortisone-like drugs directly into the bald patches. These injections are relatively painless and can hasten the regrowth, and often prevent further hair loss. In severe cases, applying cortisone-type creams to the patches and covering them tightly with plastic or Saran Wrap may help.

A topical drug, Rogaine (see page 155), also offers some promise in growing new hair in these balding patches, and your dermatologist can give you all the information regarding it.

Other treatments include PUVA, the same type of treatment that is often used to treat patients with psoriasis (see page 37), and strong sensitizing agents to stimulate the hair follicle to "switch back on." One of the latest experimental drugs for alopecia areata is one that is used in kidney transplant patients to prevent organ rejection. Called tacrolimus—Prograf—this medication has been made into an ointment that when rubbed into the balding patches might restore the hair after several weeks or months. It sounds promising, but the jury is still out…

Massage and hair tonics are worthless. If they do seem to help, it is only because time has allowed nature to do its job.

If you have an extensive and persistent case of alopecia areata, you may find that a hairpiece will give you peace of mind.

For further information regarding alopecia areata, get in touch with either of the following:
National Alopecia Areata Foundation
710 "C" Street, Suite 11
P.O. Box 150760
San Rafael, California 94915-0760
415-456-4644; Fax: 415-456-4274
E-mail: info@naaf.org
www.alopeciaareata.com

HAIR (Help Alopecia International Research)
P.O. Box 1875
Thousand Oaks, CA 91358
805-494-4903

Recap

- Patchy hair loss is pretty much like it sounds—a condition of the scalp and other hairy body areas, that begins with the appearance of one or more small, round or oval bald patches, which gradually enlarge over a period of weeks.
- The scalp is the area most commonly affected, but alopecia areata can affect the beard, eyebrows, eyelashes, and any other hairy region.
- The latest theory is that alopecia areata may be an autoimmune disorder—a type of "self- allergy," where the body rejects its own tissue, in this case the hair follicle.

EXCESS HAIR

One of the unhappiest women I know is a young lady with an excess amount of dark hair on her upper lip, her chin, and her chest. She is not alone. There are thousands of young women with the same cosmetic problem: superfluous hair; hair that doesn't look sporty in the locker room, hair where nobody wants it.

Exactly what do we mean by excess hair? Excess hair does *not* mean an increase in the number of hairs. Everyone is born with a fixed number on his or her body. This is genetically determined (inherited).

There are two types of excess hair: one, hirsutism, is the growth of excess hair in the areas of the skin, such as the face and chest, usually reserved for male hair growth. (See below.) Hypertrichosis, on the other hand, is a disorder where unwanted hair is more or less generalized in distribution. Hypertrichosis, by the way, also occurs in men.

Hair grows on every portion of the skin except the palms, soles and a few other small areas. Most are of the "peach-fuzz" variety (vellus hairs). Others are of the terminal variety—the long, thicker hairs of the scalp (think Lady Godiva and Rapunzel), the chest, and the

159

pubic region.

Excess hairiness results from the vellus hairs becoming longer, darker, and thicker in areas where one expects only peach-fuzz.

While excess hair may be due to many factors, for some groups of people it is a normal state of affairs. People from Southern Europe and Middle-Eastern cultures are much hairier than those from Northern Europe and Scandinavian countries; white people are hairier than black people; and Asians and Native Americans are the least hairy of all.

Above and beyond this normal, constitutional hairy excess are those women who exhibit a greater increase in the length and thickness of hair in certain areas usually reserved for the "peach fuzz" variety: the upper lip, the chin, the sides of the face, the areas around the nipples, and the portion of the abdomen extending from the pubic region to the belly button. (These are the areas normally associated with the male pattern hair growth.) This type of superfluous hair—hirsutism—can be especially embarrassing to the young and otherwise confident woman—one of those "thousand natural shocks that flesh is heir to."

The causes of excess hair are many and varied. For those with a moderate degree, the factors may be merely a part of normal growth and development.

The most common cause of excess hair growth in females is the aging process. Along about the time of menopause, women become deficient in the production of the female hormone estrogen. The decrease of this hormone gives rise to a relative increase in the male-type hormone (androgen), which is responsible for the proliferation of hairs thick, dark hairs appearing on the upper lip, chin, and cheeks. And at the same time begins the steady thinning of the scalp hair. These two processes seem to go hand in hand: more hair on the body, less on the scalp.

Stress can also play a role in excess hair growth. The hair follicles are under the influence of various hormones and chemicals produced by the body. Emotional stress and tension often lead to a disturbance in the delicate balance of these hormones which, in turn, can result in a stimulation of the hair follicle leading to excess hair—not, however, on the head. These hormonal imbalances also can arise in connection with tumors and cysts of the ovaries, diseases of the adrenal glands, and tumors or abnormal functioning of other hormone-secreting glands, such as the thyroid or pituitary.

In addition, various drugs and medications can occasionally produce hypertrichosis when taken over a period of time. These include drugs for epilepsy (Dilantin), cortisone-like drugs, and a host of others.

Treatment For Excess Hair

Women who have excessive hair on the body or the face can suffer deep embarrassment. It isn't a problem you get rid of by saying "presto," but there are ways of dealing with the problem.

A woman who has no hormonal disease or disturbance can conceal or remove excess hair in a number of ways: bleaching, shaving, plucking, depilatory creams and lotions, waxes, abrasive applicators, and electrolysis. All have their drawbacks and all, except electrolysis, are temporary measures.

Whether you will use any (or all) of the methods described below will depend upon the area (or areas) you intend to treat, your skin type, pain tolerance, dexterity, free time, and your pocketbook.

Bleaching: Bleaching with commercially available products can conceal excessive, fine, fuzzy hair growth on the upper lip and forearms. It is most effective for small amounts of unwanted hair.

When done properly, bleaching is simple, safe, and painless. Repeated use of bleaching agents, however, can damage the hair shaft and cause temporary breakage. It can also irritate the skin. If you do bleach and develop a rash, try a different product.

Shaving: There is a popular myth that if you shave or cut your hair, it will grow back faster, thicker, coarser, and darker. Don't believe it. There is no scientific evidence to support this old wives' tale. (If it were true, there would be very few bald men!)

The portion of hair emerging from the surface of the skin is non-living—a dead protein thread. Cutting or shaving cannot influence the growing portion of your hair—the root—that occupies the hair follicle beneath the surface of the skin. Shaving is, however, a temporary measure and one must repeat it fairly often to avoid the stub-

161

bly feel and the "5 o'clock shadow" look.

If you shave with a safety razor, I recommend a clean, sharp, single-track blade. Avoid using old, ragged blades just to get in that last use. For a good shave, wet the hair thoroughly for at least two minutes with a lather shave cream that helps prevent evaporation. Do not shave too closely, as this practice can lead to ingrown hairs. And contrary to what you may have been taught, it is advisable to shave *with* the grain, *not* against it. This will prevent ingrown hairs and subsequent infection.

If you use an electric shaver, try a preshave lotion that helps remove oil from the hair. You'll find that shaving is easier, and you'll be less likely to nick the skin.

Plucking (Tweezing): Plucking out hairs with tweezers is a popular and effective, although somewhat painful, way to remove temporarily scattered hairs on the face, chest, and eyebrows. Because of the discomfort and irritation, you should reserve this method for small areas of excess hair.

Plucking has no adverse side effects and, like other methods of temporary hair removal, will not cause the hairs to grow faster, coarser, or darker. Since the hair is removed at the root, it may grow back slower than hair that has been shaved off. Be warned, constant and repeated tweezing in the same area can cause tiny, pitted scars.

When using the plucking method, make sure the skin and the tweezers are scrupulously clean to avoid infection. Also, *do not* pluck hairs from moles, warts, or other tumors. This can cause disagreeable and dangerous side effects: bleeding, infection, and change in the type of cell growth.

Hint: to minimize pain when plucking, apply an ice cube to the area just beforehand.

Chemical Depilatories: Available in creams, liquids, and foams, these products weaken the chemical bonds of the hairs, causing them to break off or dissolve just below the surface of the skin. This is one of the best, easiest, and most popular methods for temporary removal of unwanted hair on the arms, legs, and underarm areas.

One word of caution: *do not* use these products on broken or abraded skin. It is also wise not to use them on very delicate areas, like the "bikini line" of the thighs or on the skin of the breasts.

The first time you use a chemical depilatory, try it on a "test" area first to make sure your skin isn't unusually sensitive to it. Then wash and thoroughly dry the area to be depilated. Apply the chemical and leave it on for a specific length of time—usually 10 to 15 minutes, depending on the directions given by the manufacturer. (If you leave it on longer than recommended, it can severely irritate your skin.) Rinse the area thoroughly with clear, lukewarm water, using a washcloth if necessary, and pat dry. You should then apply a soothing, emollient cream or lotion.

The main advantage of chemical depilatories is that they are painless. They also break off hairs below the surface of the skin, so regrowth is relatively slow and the hairs grow back soft, not stubbly.

Waxing: One of the oldest and least popular methods of temporary hair removal is wax. Hot, melted wax is poured onto the skin, left to cool and solidify, and then rapidly stripped off.

This type of hair removal is longer lasting than some of the other methods described. It takes about four to six weeks for waxed hair to grow back. However, there is always some degree of pain and skin irritation. Also, you cannot repeat this type of treatment until the hairs have grown out and are long enough to become embedded in the wax.

Abrasives: Pumice stones have been used for centuries to "wear off" excess hair. Although simple and inexpensive, this method of hair removal is rather tedious and uncomfortable and, therefore, not suitable for large areas.

Electrolysis: There is only one safe way to remove excess hair permanently: destroying the hair root with an electric current. This is called electrolysis.

Performed by a physician or trained electrologist, electrolysis consists of inserting a fine platinum or steel wire needle into the opening of the hair follicle. An electric current, transmitted down the needle, permanently destroys the hair root. The loosened hairs are then removed with tweezers. Once you destroy the root, the hair can no longer grow back.

While several types of electric current may be used, the basic procedure is the same. The results will depend upon the skill of the operator. Even in the most competent hands, however, electrolysis is a long, expensive, and tedious process. It is also somewhat painful, particularly on areas other than the face.

Electrolysis is most effective for the coarse, darker hairs, not the fine, "peach-fuzz," lanugo hairs. It has no effect on the cause of excessive hair growth; all it can do is destroy the existing hair.

Electrolysis is not 100 percent effective, and repeated treatments are often necessary to successfully destroy all the unwanted hairs. There are several reasons for this. Some hair follicles are bent or crooked. The electrical current for the particular follicle may be insufficient, because the higher the current, the greater the pain; therefore, the operator tries to "get away" with the smallest current that might do the job.

Also, since the electrologist works below the surface of the skin, the insertion of the needle into the hair follicle is essentially a blind procedure and cannot be performed with absolute certainty. Another common occurrence is that the hair will come out, but the papilla (the hair root) will not be destroyed, resulting in the regrowth of that particular hair. Thus, depending upon the skill of the operator and nature of the hair, a single strand may have to be treated several times before it stops growing.

Coarse hairs may return three or four times, but these become finer at each regrowth. Eventually the root is so effectively destroyed that the hairs can no longer grow.

"Sittings" with the electrologist should be no longer than half an hour, during which time only a limited number of hairs, about fifty, should be removed. To avoid excessive irritation, hairs lying close together should not be dealt with at the same time. Also, the skin and needles must be adequately sterilized to prevent infection.

In the hands of a competent, well-trained electrologist the dangers and side effects are minimal. Occasionally, scarring and fine pits will develop in places formerly occupied by hairs. One sees this more commonly on the upper lip, therefore it is best to avoid treatment on this area.

Excessive pigmentation may develop, but this is rare and usually quickly disappears. Since it is impossible to predict the nature of scarring or healing in any given patient, the electrologist should try a trial area first and check the results.

I do not recommend the small, battery-operated, do-it-yourself kits. It is virtually impossible for a person to insert a tiny needle into a hair follicle on his or her face—while looking in a mirror! And when improperly used, these self-treatments can lead to irreparable scarring.

If you are contemplating electrolysis, don't expect too much. The average patient quickly tires of the experience and the cost. Because only a small percentage of hairs can be removed at one sitting, and because some regrowth of hair—even in the most skilled hands—will always recur, it requires firm dedication on the part of you and the operator. A severe case of excess hair (hirsutism) may require years of treatment. But despite its limitations, in selected patients electrolysis is useful and successful.

Several new *laser treatments* appear to be effective in removing unwanted hair. Many dermatologists have availed themselves of this method. Again, check with your dermatologist to find out if he or she does this procedure, or if a referral to a laser-hair specialist will be in order. There are a variety of lasers that will do the job, and several of these go by the following names: Nd:YAG, Long Pulse Ruby, Long Pulse Alexandrite, and Diode.

Other than these physical and mechanical methods are some oral medications that seem to influence and control excessive hair growth:

- High-dose oral contraceptive pills. With their high estrogen levels, these suppress the amount of androgens (male-type hormone) in the ovaries, and act to slow down this objectionable hair production.
- Cimetidine (Tagamet)—a drug used for stomach ulcers. This drug affects male hormone production and also checks excess hair growth.
- Spironolactone—a medication used for high blood pressure. This also works as an anti-androgen, and by suppressing androgenic activity in the skin, inhibits the growth of unwanted hair.
- Dexamethasone—a cortisone-like drug. This drug suppresses the adrenal gland, and some doctors consider this to be the best treatment for hypertrichosis.

These oral medications are still in the experimental stages. Your dermatologist can give you further information about them.

The very latest method for the treatment of excess hair is a topical drug called Vaniqa (eflornithine). Approved by the Food and Drug Administration in the fall of 2000, Vaniqa is believed to work by blocking an enzyme necessary for hair growth, thus slowing the rate of re-growth of excessive facial hair in women. The results seem to be impressive, but before considering this prescription medication, do check with your dermatologist. It should be stressed that Vaniqa is *not* a depilatory (hair remover); it supplements current methods of hair removal. One has to be patient with this method. Results may not be noticeable for several weeks.

For further information about excess hair, log on to www.aad.org
1-888-462-DERM x22
or www.familydoctor.org/handouts/210.html

Recap

- Excess hairiness results from the "peach-fuzz" hairs becoming longer, darker, and thicker in areas where one expects to have only peach-fuzz.
- Emotional stress and tension often lead to a disturbance in the delicate balance of various hormones which, in turn, can result in a stimulation of the hair follicle leading to excess hair—not, however, on the head.
- There is only one safe way to remove excess hair permanently: destroying the hair root with an electric current. This is called electrolysis.

A FEW NOTES ON SHAVING

The average adult male has about 30,000 hairs on his face and it has been estimated that he will shave away about 30 feet of beard during a lifetime of shaving.

The growth of the beard varies with the time of day: more growth during the day than at night with the most rapid growth occurring around the age of thirty.

The rate of beard growth—like other hairy areas—is not affected by shaving or by any other method of removal.

Most men with dark beards believe that theirs are heavier than those of men who have light hair. This is erroneous. While the dark color is more readily noticed, the color of hair is not related to the density.

If you have any problems with shaving, here are a few tips to make the process smoother and less irritating:

- To soften the hairs, wash your face thoroughly with soap and hot water for at least two minutes. Rinse.
- Apply an aerosol shaving cream and lather up for two more minutes.
- Use only a single-edge, disposable razor.
- Shave gently, using smooth, even strokes.
- Shave down—one way—on the cheeks and chin.
- Shave up—one way—on the neck.
- Shave over one area only one time. *Do not* shave repeatedly over the same area.
- Don't pull your beard taut when shaving.
- Use a new razor blade every time you shave. If you can find a single-edge disposable razor, use it.
- Shave every other day for the first two weeks, then daily.

6 Nails and Nail Disorders

NAILS

Just think: if you didn't have fingernails, how would you open your birthday presents, untie your shoelaces, button your shirt, peel off labels, or pull tacks out of bulletin boards? A variety of simple, everyday tasks would be difficult or impossible without fingernails.

You couldn't pluck guitar strings, pick up coins or take off earrings. It would be pretty challenging to open flip-top cans, peel oranges, or separate *Life Savers* that are stuck together. And, thanks to nails, you can scratch where it itches.

Our twenty nails are pretty important, and though we neglect and abuse them, they serve us for a lifetime. And we spend more than $500-million a year to keep them beautiful and "healthy" even though our nails are actually dead.

Once the human's only tools, the function of nails has changed in the course of evolution. In lower animals, nails—as sharp claws or strong hooves—serve for protection, locomotion, climbing and eating.

Historically, they have been a means of personal decoration. Long nails, often accented by jeweled fingertip extenders, were a mark of the leisure class in Asian cultures for many centuries. Growing up to a foot long, they were the sign of a life of complete idleness. Even today, well-manicured nails can be a status symbol. Some salons offer gold tips and diamond studs.

Although our nails have now become relatively weak and flat, they still serve many useful functions:

- They protect the tips of our fingers and toes from injury and foreign substances.
- They aid the fingertips in our sense of touch.
- They help us grasp small objects and use our fingers more efficiently. This is important in delicate mechanical work.
- They help in defense and attack.
- They are used for scratching.
- They can serve as a mirror of our general state of health. Problems with our nails can be an indication of an internal disease.

What exactly are nails?

Made up of a protein called keratin, nails are specialized horny extensions of our skin. This protein has a high amount of sulfur and it's the sulfur that makes the nails hard and rigid. (For added strength, nails are curved in both directions.) The keratin of our nails is similar to the keratin that makes up our hair. Nails and hair have many things in common:

- Both have their beginnings deep inside the skin. Both are dead, so that they can be cut or trimmed painlessly. And since they aren't living, there's nothing you can put on them to make them grow any better, faster, longer, stronger, or thicker.
- Both depend upon the body's processes and a rich blood supply for nourishment and growth. Both can regenerate. If you pluck a hair out of your head, it grows back normally; if you lose a nail, it usually grows back normally as well.

Nails consist of several structures: (see Figure)

1. The nail plate. The visible part of the nail on the fingers and toes. This is what we mean when we refer to our "nail." It's firmly attached to the nail bed underneath.
2. The nail bed. The skin beneath the nail plate. This network of capillaries supplies the blood and gives the pinkish color to the nail plate.
3. The nail matrix. This is the most important structure of our nail;

170

it is the hidden part of the nail unit where growth takes place. Made up of living cells that produce the nail plate, it is located beneath the cuticle. If this matrix is damaged, the nail will be distorted.

4. The lunula. The visible part of the matrix is called the lunula or "half moon"—the small, lighter-colored arc you usually see on your thumbs and big toes. The shape of the end of your nail plate depends on the shape of your half moons.

5. The cuticle. The cuticle is the fold of skin at the base of the nail plate. Made up of dead cells, it seals the skin to the nail to keep foreign substances from working their way into the narrow space between the skin and the nail.

6. Nail folds. The folds of skin that support the nail on three sides.

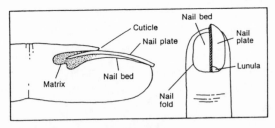

Nails will grow indefinitely if not cut or injured. They grow at different rates for everyone, depending on each person's state of health. It takes about five months for a fingernail to grow from the cuticle to the end of your fingertip. It takes longer for a thumbnail and twice as long for toenails.

Here are some other trivia to nail you with:

- Nails grow faster in summer than in winter, faster during the day than at night, faster in men than in women, and faster in children than in adults.
- Nail growth slows down as we get older, and nails tend to thicken and become irregular.
- The middle fingernail grows the fastest, and the pinkie nail the slowest.
- If you are right-handed, your nails grow faster on the right hand and vice versa.

- Nails grow faster in nail-biters, typists, and piano players, which is convenient since they use them up faster!
- They grow faster in women who are premenstrual and who are in the early stages of pregnancy.
- Starvation diets slow down the growth of nails.
- Gelatin has absolutely no value in treating nail problems.

Despite what the horror movies would make you believe, nails do not grow after death. What seems like continued nail growth is only the drying and shrinking of the soft tissues around the nail plates.

We used to believe that the hardness of nails, like bones and teeth, was the result of their calcium content. Actually, there's very little calcium in the nail plate, not enough to make a difference. So taking calcium supplements won't help soft nails.

"Healthy" Nails and Nail Care

Actually, there is no such thing as a healthy nail. Since the nail plate is dead, it can't really be healthy. But there are a variety of diseases and disorders that can affect the characteristics of your nails.

Everyone longs for healthy-*looking* nails, smooth and neatly trimmed. Healthy-looking nails have no grooves, ridges, or pits and no spots or discolorations. Nails, by nature, are hard and strong. But, like the skin and other body organs, they should be treated with gentle care.

Here are a few guidelines to help you grow, and keep, healthy-looking, attractive nails:

- Since nails are easier to cut when they're soft, soak them in warm water for about 30 minutes before cutting and trimming. File them when they're dry.
- Don't overuse polishes, base coats and polish remover. They can cause nail problems and irritate your skin.
- Remove hangnails with clean, sharp scissors. Pulling or biting them can lead to infection.
- Treat your cuticles gently. Be careful when using cuticle-removing solutions since they can destroy tissue when left on too long. If you want to push back your cuticles, first soak your fingertips in warm water for about 20 minutes and then gently push them back using

an orange stick. Remember that your cuticle is there for a purpose—to protect your nail. Tampering with it opens the door to harmful germs and infection. It's a better idea just to leave your cuticles alone. If you wear rubber gloves, even the cotton-lined variety, always wear soft, cotton liners (Dermal gloves) inside them. When your hands are in hot water, they sweat and react with the chemicals from the rubber, plastic or vinyl in the gloves.

This can cause problems for your skin and nails. A recent newspaper article warns of salon footbaths when having pedicures. Boils and ulcers of the toes in many women developed apparently from a microbe growing in a footbath used for pedicures.

- When gardening or doing other heavy work, protect your nails by wearing canvas gloves.
- To prevent chipping, peeling and tearing, and to keep your nails flexible, moisturize them. Soak them in water for 20 minutes and then apply an emollient cream, such as Elta or Cutemol.
- To strengthen nails, tap them—on desks, tabletops and other surfaces.
- Do not use your nails as a screwdriver, can opener, pliers, or telephone dialer (not a problem with push-button phones).
- To prevent ingrown toenails, cut them straight across, so that the edges of the nail don't poke into the skin folds along the sides.
- Keep nails clean and dry to prevent bacteria and fungi from collecting under the nail.

Nail Cosmetics

Decorating the nails is a universal practice that's been around since the beginning of time. Today, there are dozens of products and preparations to decorate, as well as protect and repair them.

We have nail enamels, varnishes and lacquers; top coats, base coats and undercoats; nail conditioners, hardeners and whiteners; buffing creams; enamel removers and cuticle removers; cuticle creams and oils; pre-formed, plastic and gold press-on nails; sculptured and porcelain nail extenders; nail mending and nail wrapping kits.

While some of these products can make nails more resistant to damage, all of them could possibly cause irritation and allergic reactions. The dyes in nail polish can cause rashes on your eyelids, face, neck, upper chest, and even in the anal and genital areas—but almost never around your nails. The glues, resins and formaldehyde found in many nail products can irritate the nail plate and surrounding tissues and result in brittleness, discoloration, pain, lifting up of the nail, and infection.

Nail Disorders

The condition of your nails, like that of your skin and hair, depends on your general health. When your body suffers from infection, disease or dietary deficiency, the growth, texture and appearance of your nails can change.

The most common nail problems are caused by fungous infections, psoriasis, lichen planus, pigmentation, and allergies to nail cosmetics.

Sudden and serious physical stress, as from a tragic accident or a major surgical operation, may dramatically change the pattern of your nail growth. This happens because nail growth is expendable, which means your body ignores it under severe stress. The growth of your nails may slow down temporarily or stop altogether. Weeks after your health has improved, you'll be able to see transverse ridges on all your nails, reflecting the period when growth was interrupted. Other changes in your nails can foretell, among other factors, illness, injury, or poor nail care.

Onycholysis is a separation of the nail (plate) from the nail bed. It is often associated with yeast and fungal infections, from nail cosmetics—base coats, frosted nail polish, topcoats—or injury due to improper manicuring, thyroid, diabetes, and a variety of internal disorders. Many medications can also cause onycholysis.

Brittle nails are nails that have lost their strength. They split, chip, crack and break off easily. Brittleness is usually due to harsh household products, strong soaps and detergents, glues, cleaning solvents, furniture polish, and irritating and allergenic nail cosmetics (polish, removers, hardeners, etc.).

The weather can also cause brittleness. When the relative humidity is very low, the water content of the nail is decreased, making the nail more rigid and likely to fracture.

174

Finally, brittle and fragile nails can be a result of a protein deficiency, crash dieting, some illnesses, and skin diseases, as well as the aging process.

Nails can also develop *ridges*. These irregular bumps can either run along the nail's length (longitudinal) or horizontally across the nail (transverse).

Longitudinal ridges are often related to an anemic condition. Transverse ridges are usually caused by an inflammation of the skin around the nail due to skin diseases such as eczema and allergic dermatitis, or sometimes by an injury that stops the growth of the nail.

Another common condition is *thickening of the nail*. This happens on the toenails when you let them grow too long or wear tight shoes that cramp their growth. Thick nails are also associated with flat feet, obesity, and fungous infections.

Pitting and stippling of the nails results from a defect in the growth center (matrix) of the nail. These small indentations on the nail plate are often seen in people who have psoriasis, eczema or alopecia areata.

Thinning of the nails happens with anemia, thyroid disorders and protein deficiency in crash-dieters.

Spoon-shaped depressions in the nails can be a sign of anemia, as well as thyroid and other hormonal disorders.

Separation of the nail plate from the nail bed is a common condition. Each time you clean under your nail with a fingernail file or a toothpick, you cause a tiny separation between the nail plate and the nail bed. Repeated cleanings cause a dead space to form where moisture and germs collect and grow. The nail bed becomes infected, the nail plate separates from the bed, and the color underneath the nail changes from pink to yellow, green or black, depending on which germ has set up housekeeping.

Sometimes this results from too much time with your hands in soap and water, as well as from injury, certain drugs, fungous infections, psoriasis, and thyroid disorders.

Pigmented (discolored) nails occur for a variety of reasons. Nails can become permanently stained from heavy smoking, and working with inks, shoe polishes, dyes and chemicals. Nail injuries and tight shoes can make your nails turn black, due to bleeding beneath the affected nails. For example, athletes in track and field events, joggers, dancers, and tennis and racquetball players can develop blackened toenails from repeatedly jamming their feet into the front of their shoes.

Certain diseases can affect the color of the nails. A patient with yellow nails, for example, should be evaluated for some systemic disease. A diffuse, bright red color may develop in patients with cardiac disease.

Fungal and bacterial infections, diabetes, and certain lung, liver and kidney diseases can change the color of your nails. So can antibiotics, anticancer medication, sulfa, and other drugs. Lithium can induce a number of nail changes, including the appearance of transverse brown bands.

White spots are often seen on the nails as a result of rough manicuring, typing, filing and nail biting, as well as from nutritional deficiency, fungous infections, thyroid conditions, and anemia.

Nail *breakage* can occur from using the nails as handy tools. Nails are strong, but not as strong as screwdrivers, can openers, and pliers.

Clubbing—a bulbous enlargement at the end of the fingers with exaggerated curvatures of the nail—is associated with several systemic diseases, notably congestive heart failure, emphysema, cirrhosis, and a variety of internal malignant tumors.

Paronychia is an infection or inflammation around the nail folds caused by bacteria or fungous germs. It can result from a nail injury, nail biting, and from keeping your hands in water for a long time. It's a common problem for bartenders, waitresses and housewives (and househusbands).

Ingrown nails are a common nail problem, particularly on the big toes. This painful condition is often a result of tight shoes, improper nail trimming, or injury that causes a corner of the nail to turn downwards into the skin. An ingrown nail requires the attention of a dermatologist before infection sets in.

Fungal infections of the toenails make up about half of all nail disorders in the adult. Toenails are affected more often than fingernails because they are confined in a warm, moist environment where they proliferate.

Warts often occur around and beneath the nail folds. They can

176

be very difficult to treat, but a special method (see page 31) may get rid of them quickly and painlessly.

Treatment of Nail Disorders

The treatment of nail disorders will depend upon the type of problem you have and what's causing it. Try to figure out and get rid of what you think might be responsible for the condition. Correct any general disorder or disease you may have, and eat a well-balanced diet.

For a continuing and stubborn nail problem, see your dermatologist. Remember, nails can be mirrors of other, more serious health problems.

For further information about nail health, log on to:
www.aad.org
1-888-462-DERM x22

Recap

- Our twenty nails are pretty important, and though we neglect and abuse them, they serve us for a lifetime.
- Made up of a protein called keratin, nails are specialized horny extensions of our skin. This protein has a high amount of sulfur, which makes the nails hard and rigid.
- It takes about five months for a fingernail to grow from the cuticle to the end of your fingertip. It takes longer for a thumbnail and twice as long for toenails.
- Brittle and fragile nails can be a result of a protein deficiency, crash dieting, some illnesses and skin diseases, as well as the aging process.

7
Black Skin and Hair Conditions

For openers, let me state that black skin is firmer, stronger, and smoother than white skin and is much more resistant to photo-damage and the aging process. A recent study comparing forty- to fifty-year-old white women's skin to those of African-American women revealed that nearly all the white women in the study had definite wrinkles, "crow's feet," on the corners of the mouth and eyes, while the black women had very few.

Black people, however, are troubled by unique skin problems. Also, their skin reacts differently to injury and various ailments.

Some skin disorders are more common—and more apparent—in black people: keloids, "razor bumps," vitiligo, lupus erythematosus, tinea versicolor, acne due to pomades applied to the scalp, "ashy skin," pityriasis alba, and others. Some diseases of the skin are considered unusual or rare among black people: scabies, head lice, and rosacea are some examples of these uncommon ailments.

Many skin problems in blacks are related to cosmetics designed for use on black skin, and to fashion trends that are more common among blacks. For example, the use of creams and oils to reduce ashy skin color can cause hair follicle infections of the body and scalp. Also, cornrowing, hot combing, and hair-straightening chemicals often lead to scalp irritation and temporary hair loss.

Some allergies seem to show up more frequently in black people as well. The most common cause of allergic reactions in black

179

women is an ingredient called paraphenylenediamine, used in hair dyes. Allergies to nickel can cause a rash on the earlobes from earrings and on the ears and temples from the nickel in eyeglass frames. Black men have a tendency to develop severe and continuing allergies to chromium compounds in cement and leather. Because of the scratching and rubbing that goes along with allergy rashes, black skin usually thickens and develops excess pigmentation, which can become a cosmetic problem.

Care of Black Skin

While its true that black skin is stronger, has the physiological advantage of resisting sun damage, and doesn't show its age as easily as white skin, it doesn't mean you don't have to take good care of it. To keep black skin healthy-looking, and to prevent the excess pigmentation that can develop on troubled and inflamed skin, follow these guidelines:

- Don't use abrasive cleansers on your face.
- Don't use harsh detergent soaps.
- Do not squeeze pimples.
- Do not use Vaseline or pomades on your scalp or face.
- Try not to scratch or irritate your skin.

Let's look at some of the skin and hair conditions that are common to black people.

SKIN CONDITIONS

Pigmentation Problems

Problems with skin pigment or color—too much or too little—can be a real concern if you're black. They show up more and are more apparent because of the stronger contrast between the normal and problem skin. They also last longer than pigmentary problems in less dark skin.

Even though this may sound strange, people of *all* races have the *same number* of color-producing cells in their skin. These cells are called melanocytes. The melanocytes in black skin produce more color or pigment, and make it faster, than white skin. Furthermore, they are larger, more active, and circulated differently from those in white skin. (See chapter on Pigmentation.) Because of this, pigmentary changes in black people are usually more obvious and longer lasting. The advantage of black skin is twofold: blacks rarely, if ever, develop skin cancer and they do not show the aging changes—wrinkles—as readily as whites.

Many of the color variations in black skin are normal. For example, black skin is lighter on the palms of the hands and soles of the feet, and darker on the gums, the roof of the mouth, and the inner surfaces of the cheeks. Black people often have brown or black stripes on the nails of the thumb and index finger as well as lines of pigmentation on the upper arms.

Excessive pigmentation in black skin can be the result of a simple injury, a mild irritation, or from diseases such as acne or eczema. This extra- or *hyper*pigmentation indicates increased activity of the color-producing cells when the skin is injured or inflamed. It can last for months or years, which can be very distressing.

Hyperpigmentation is often seen in young black people who are being treated for acne. Blacks usually have a reaction to the drying and peeling medications used in acne therapy. The discoloration can last for years while the patient is using lotions and creams that contain the drying ingredients.

Other skin disorders that can cause color variations in black skin are eczema, psoriasis, lichen planus, tinea versicolor, and pityriasis rosea. These same conditions, paradoxically, can cause a loss of pigment or *hypo*pigmentation. Skin injuries and liquid nitrogen treatments used to treat warts and other tumors can also cause pigmentary changes.

While there is no easy cure for these annoying pigmentary changes, you can help some of them with cortisone-like creams and ointments, which your dermatologist will be able to prescribe. Other methods include some over-the-counter preparations that are discussed in the chapter on Pigment Disorders (see page 189).

Ashy Skin

Ashy skin is simply dry skin. It is a result of the body getting rid of dead skin cells. This normal shedding happens in all races. Grayish, ashy-looking skin shows up more clearly on black skin because of the contrast between the dead, dry cells on the surface and the fresh, new ones that have replaced them. It's *not* a sign of disease.

You can take care of this perfectly normal, healthy skin very easily, using the same treatment as for dry skin (see page 42.) Wash with a mild, gentle soap or skin cleanser (like Cetaphil Cleanser), bathe in Alpha Keri Oil, apply a moisturizer (like Cetaphil Lotion) after your bath, and try to increase the relative humidity in your home to at least 40 percent.

Avoid the use of greasy and oily products—cocoa butter, cold creams, petroleum jelly—to attempt to alleviate this condition. Such products will only plug up your oil glands and lead to acne bumps on your face and other areas.

Lichenification

Black skin appears to be especially susceptible to developing lichenification. This harmless condition consists of thickened, hyperpigmented patches of skin with accentuated skin markings. It is a result of constant scratching that accompanies eczema, contact dermatitis, and some types of "nervous" itching. People who are under constant stress often develop itchy areas—back of neck, forearms, legs and ankles, and other areas—that they (naturally) scratch and rub. This persistent scratching and rubbing will bring on thickening and darkening.

Pityriasis Alba

This common condition occurs primarily in childhood—ages eight to twelve usually—and is a marker of eczema. Although it also occurs in white children, it is more noticeable in black skin. It consists of light—*hypo*pigmented—patches of skin over the cheeks, and, occasionally other areas such as the arms and neck. It also has another name—furfuraceous impetigo—but rest assured, it has nothing to do with impetigo (see page 122).

Dermatosis Papulosa Nigra

Dermatosis papulosa nigra is a condition, not a disease, seen

182

almost exclusively in blacks. It occurs in about one-third of all black people and is twice as common in women as in men.

What does it look like? Tiny, smooth, raised, mole-like spots that appear on the face and neck, which are darker than the skin around them. Resembling flat warts, they begin around the age of puberty, are inherited, can vary in number from a few to hundreds, and increase in number as a person gets older. They never become malignant; in other words, they are not precancerous growths. Some of the well-known people who have these growths are Maya Angelou, Bill Cosby and Morgan Freeman.

If you have a lot of these tumors and are unhappy with the way they look, a dermatologist can remove them simply and easily through a variety of methods.

HAIR AND SCALP CONDITIONS

Hair Loss and Hair Breakage

The woolly, kinky texture of black hair is uniquely different in its shape and structure from the soft, straight, flowing hair of white or Asian people.

Hair-grooming procedures such as curling, pressing and perming stretch and stress the hair, causing it to break off or fall out.

Traction alopecia is a term used to describe symmetrical hair loss at the margins of the hairline. In other words, a receding hairline. This condition can result from tightly braided or twisted hairstyles, tight rollers and heated curlers, as well as decorative cornrowing and dreadlocks. These can cause permanent hair loss.

Using a hot comb on chemically treated hair can result in hair loss over the crown or top of the head.

Using chemical relaxers and hair straighteners improperly or too frequently can cause patchy baldness by damaging the keratin of the hair, making it brittle and easy to break off.

Using a pick can fracture the hair shaft, also leading to hair loss.

To prevent or manage hair loss and breakage, ease the stress on your hair. This may mean changing your hairstyle, wearing looser braids, or using pin curls instead of rollers. Also, make sure you shampoo your hair at least once a week (I know it's often difficult), and use a protein conditioner regularly.

"Razor Bumps"

The ingrown hairs of the beard in black men are called, technically, pseudofolliculitis barbae. Almost everyone knows what you mean, though, if you call them "razor bumps."

This irritation and swelling around an ingrown hair occurs mostly in young black men because the hair and hair follicles in blacks are more curved than in whites.

Razor bumps develop when the sharp, razor-cut tips of curly hair, sharpened by frequent shaving, cut into the skin in an arc and grow inward. [See Figure A.] Because of the natural curve of the hair follicles of African-Americans, the hair grows like a curved needle and grows back into the skin. This induces a reaction called a "foreign body reaction:" redness, swelling and pain.

Several factors make the condition worse:

- Stretching the skin out and pulling it taut when shaving. Once the skin is released, the short hairs pull back below the surface of the skin. Because of their curve and sharp tip, they reenter the skin and pierce the wall of the hair follicle.
- Shaving against the grain.
- Shaving with a dull blade.
- Shaving with a 2-track razor. That extra track cuts the hair below the level of the skin before it has a chance to snap back.

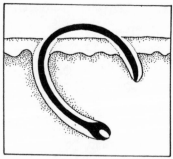

Figure A

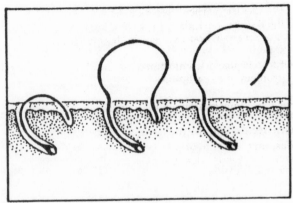

Figure B

There are no easy solutions to this common, painful inconvenience, but here are a few hints that can help:

- The simplest answer is to grow a beard and all the bumps will disappear in about a month. Why? Because by the time the hairs are about a half-inch long (in a month or so), the natural tension will cause the ends of the hairs to spring out of the skin. [See Figure B.]
- Since you may not want a beard for the rest of your life, change your shaving routine as follows:

1. Before shaving, carefully lift out any ingrown hairs with a straight pin or a beard pick onto the skin surface. Do not pluck them out! (See #12 below.)
2. To soften the hairs, wash your face vigorously with soap and hot water, using a face cloth, for at least two minutes. Rinse.
3. Apply an aerosol shaving cream and lather up for two more minutes.
4. Use only a single-edge razor.
5. Shave gently, using smooth, even strokes.
6. Shave down—one way—on the cheeks and chin.
7. Shave up—one way—on the neck.
8. Shave over one area only one time. **Do not** shave repeatedly over the same area.
9. Don't pull your beard taut when shaving.
10. Use a new razor blade every time you shave. If you can find a single-edge disposable razor, use it.

11. Shave every other day for the first two weeks, then daily.

12. Inspect for trapped hairs at night. Clean these with alcohol, and then flick these hairs onto the skin surface. **Do not pluck them out!** Leave them until morning at which time they will appear on the surface of the skin.

Don't expect to get a smooth, clean shave the first few times you use this method. Be patient. After a while, you may be able to train your hairs to grow out straight, or at least straighter, rather than in a curl.

If this method doesn't work, here are a few other suggestions:

- Use a chemical depilatory. But beware—they can be irritating, they take a long time to use, they don't smell very pleasant, and they should not be used more often than every other day.
- Use electric barber clippers to shave. Since they cut the hair less short, they do prevent razor bumps. At the same time, though, you may not be happy with a less close shave.
- Electric shavers, unfortunately, aren't much help with the problem of razor bumps.

The latest treatment for this troublesome and stubborn condition is with a special type of laser (the long-pulsed Nd:YAG laser). Ask your dermatologist about this new, promising remedy.

For further information about black skin, log on to www.aad.org
1-888-462-DERM x22
For more information about " razor bumps," write to:
PFB Project (Pseudofolliculitis Barbae)
4801 Massachusetts Avenue, NW, Suite 400
Washington, DC 20016-2087
202-364-8710

Recap

- Black people are troubled by unique skin problems. Also, their skin reacts differently to injury and various ailments.
- Many skin problems in blacks are related to cosmetics designed for use on black skin and to fashion trends that are more common among blacks.

- Ashy-looking skin shows up more clearly on black skin because of the contrast between the dead, dry cells on the surface and the fresh, new ones that have replaced them. It's *not* a sign of disease.
- "Razor bumps" develop when the sharp, razor-cut tips of curly hair, sharpened by frequent shaving, cut into the skin in an arc and grow inward.

8
Pigment Disorders

Normal skin color, an important part of everyone's life, is dependent upon the amount and size of certain pigment granules in the upper layers of the skin. This basic skin color is determined at birth and cannot be altered.

All human skin contains three important pigments:

1. Melanin: this black pigment in your skin is produced by special pigment cells called melanocytes. All of us—black, yellow, red, and white—*have the same number of these melanocytes in our skin*, approximately 60,000 per square inch.

Then why aren't we all black?

Racial and ethnic variations in skin color depend on the size and shape of these melanocytes, the amount of melanin they produce, the speed at which the pigment is formed, the manner in which this pigment is concentrated in the skin, and the color of the melanin, which can vary from light tan to black.

Melanin is produced in the skin as small, insoluble granules. Where there are no melanin granules, the skin is white; the more melanin granules, the darker the skin. The variations in your particular skin color—tan, brown, black—will depend upon the concentration of these granules in your epidermis.

In black people, melanin production is evenly distributed, producing uniform skin color. In redheads, and in some blonds with blue eyes, melanin is produced in clumps, resulting in splotchy pigmentation—freckles.

Freckles, probably the most common pigmentary alteration in the skin, first appears at about the age of six as flat, light-brown, pigmented spots over sun-exposed skin. During the summer, they have a tendency to increase in number, size, and darkness.

The depth of the melanin granules will also affect the color of your skin: the deeper the granules, the more your skin will take on a bluish cast.

2. Hemoglobin: this pigment is responsible for giving red blood cells their color. If you are anemic, your skin will be pale; if you have too much hemoglobin, your skin will take on a ruddy complexion.

3. Carotene: this pigment, which gives your skin a yellowish cast, comes from outside the body, and is dependent upon what you eat. A diet consisting of large amounts of oranges, carrots, and squash can be responsible for an orange-yellow staining of the skin.

Excessive Pigmentation

The most common cause of excessive pigmentation is an increased stimulation in the production of melanin due to certain hormonal changes, sun exposure, or a combination of both. This condition, called melasma, appears as a dark, splotchy, brownish pigmentation on the face that develops slowly and fades with time. It usually affects women but occasionally is seen in young men who use aftershave lotions, scented soaps, and other toiletries.

Melasma is especially common in young white women, who often develop this blotchiness on their foreheads, cheeks, and mustache areas. It occurs frequently during pregnancy and is more common in brunettes than in blonds. Often called "the mask of pregnancy," melasma is more pronounced in summer due to sun exposure, and usually fades a few months after delivery. Repeated pregnancies, however, often increase the intensity of this pigmentation.

Melasma also occurs as a side effect of taking the higher-dose birth control pills. It may also be noted in apparently healthy, normal, nonpregnant women due to some mild and harmless hormonal imbalance.

Sun exposure, following the use of deodorant soaps, scented toiletries, and various cosmetics, can also produce this mottled pigmentation. This is what we call a phototoxic reaction; it is due to ultraviolet radiation being absorbed by the chemical substance (perfume, cologne, and other types of fragrance) on the skin. This pigmentation often extends to the sun-exposed areas of the neck and may be more pronounced on the left side of the forehead, face, and neck due to sun exposure while driving a car.

Excess pigmentation can also be triggered by injury to the skin (burns, abrasions, bruises), by inflammatory disorders (acne, eczema, contact dermatitis, pityriasis rosea, lichen planus) of the skin particularly in dark-skinned people, by X-rays, and by heat.

Treating Excessive Pigmentation

How can you treat excessive pigmentation of the skin?

- Above all, protect those pigmented areas from sunlight by using a high-powered sunscreen.
- Protect the areas from irritation: no strong soaps, no abrasive cleansers, no Buf-Pufs, no loofah pads. Use only a mild, gentle soap for washing.
- Try one of the over-the-counter bleaching creams that contain hydroquinone and use only as directed. Ironically, some of these can cause further pigmentation if they are too strong for your particular skin.

  If these don't work, try bleaching creams with a higher percent of hydroquinone, which are by prescription only. Some of the newer ones that work nicely are Glyquin, Lustra and Melanex.
- A good home remedy is fresh lemon juice. Cut a fresh lemon in half and squeeze the juice into a small dish. With a Q-Tip or cotton ball, gently rub the patches twice daily. Use it for at least six weeks, at which time you may see a lightening.

With any local, over-the-counter product, you must remember to be patient; it may take months before you notice any appreciable fading. Occasionally, your dark areas may fade away even without treatment.

If you believe that your pigmentation is a result of taking birth control pills, try to switch to a lower-dose type with the approval of your doctor or, if possible, stop them altogether.

If none of these treatments work, your dermatologist can try a variety of methods to eliminate these pigmented areas:

- Freezing them off gently with liquid nitrogen.
- Applying either phenol or trichloroacetic acid.
- Prescribing topical retinoic acid (Retin-A) along with a strong hydroquinone cream.
- Desiccate them lightly with an electric needle.
- Chemical peels.
- A recent alternative is the carbon dioxide and Erbium:YAG lasers.

If your condition does not respond to any type of treatment, or while waiting for the dark areas to disappear, you can mask them with a cover-up such as Covermark or Dermablend.

Above all, try to be patient...

Liver Spots

The so-called "liver spots" are nothing more than flat patches of excess pigmentation associated with sun exposure and the aging process. (They have nothing to do with the liver.) They are often called "age spots," and are extremely common in white people, beginning in their sixties. They appear over the backs of the hands, the face and forearms—the areas of the greatest amount of sun exposure. It is interesting to note that these pigment changes (as well as keratoses and skin cancers) occur in the United States more on the left side of sun-exposed areas.

The sun that shines in the window on the driver's side allows longwave ultraviolet light to penetrate the glass. That results in sun-induced problems, particularly for those who drive automobiles. In England, Australia and other countries, where the driver maneuvers the car from the right side, the reverse is true.

Since these are benign lesions, no treatment is required. But for cosmetic reasons they can be eradicated with a variety of methods. Topical treatments include fresh lemon juice (see Home Remedies section), freezing them off with liquid nitrogen by a dermatologist, chemical peels, the topical application of bleaching or fading creams, or by applying some of the so-called, over-the-counter AHAs (alpha-hydroxy acids) or Retin-A.

To protect yourself from developing these sun-induced skin changes, avoid fragrances when in the sun, use a sunscreen at all times, and wear a hat.

Dark Circles Under Eyes

This, the number two problem for women after wrinkles, is an age-old dilemma and an age-old question: Why do "bags" and dark circles occur in certain people? Truthfully, no one knows the answer! There are many theories and speculation why they develop. Here are a few of them, none of which have any valid basis or proof:

- It is hereditary. That is my guess. If you have ever seen pictures of Anne Frank, you may have noted the extremely dark circles under her pretty, brown eyes. I have been to Anne Frank's house in Amsterdam several times and have noted some of the photos of her relatives on the walls: almost all of whom had those same dark circles.
- They are worse in people who smoke.
- They are more prevalent in people with allergies (this may be a result of rubbing the eyes more than usual). They are common in people with eczema (see page 32) who, when they scratch, cause a swelling of all four eyelids.
- The skin of the eyelids is very thin. This causes the blood vessels to become more visible and noticeable, giving your lower eyelids a darker appearance.
- Dark circles of the eyelids can be a result of swelling of the lower eyelids.
- Fatigue and loss of sleep. These certainly can aggravate the conditions.
- Pregnancy.

Treatments for the dark circles are concealers and, possibly, topical vitamin K. One thing that is certain: dark circles and bags do not indicate any illness in the body.

Treatment for bags is plastic surgery. No topical measures will work.

Vitiligo—Loss of Pigmentation

Vitiligo is a mysterious malady characterized by a gradual or rapid loss of pigment, or skin color. If affects about one out of every hundred people and is more common among younger individuals. Approximately half the people who develop this ailment suffer some pigment loss before the age of twenty.

No one knows what triggers this strange condition. The most fashionable theory claims that it is one of the autoimmune disorders in which the body attacks and destroys its own tissues—in this case the pigment producing cells. We *do* know that it results from a decrease or loss of the normal cells (melanocytes) that are responsible for the production of pigment (melanin) in the skin. If the melanocytes are unable to produce melanin, or if their number decreases, white, sharply-bordered patches of different shapes and sizes will develop on otherwise normal skin.

Vitiligo can occur on any portion of the skin surface where pigment cells are present, but more commonly involves the exposed parts—the face, neck, and backs of the hands. There is no way to predict how much pigment a person will lose. In severe cases the loss of pigment can extend over the entire body. The hairs in these depigmented patches also turn white. When the pigment returns, it happens in and around these hairs first.

The pattern of vitiligo is unclear, although the condition appears to run in families. Most of the people afflicted are in good health. Occasionally, however, vitiligo occurs in association with such conditions as pernicious anemia, thyroid disease, diabetes, and disorders of the adrenal glands. Some cases follow sunburn or severe emotional stress. If you do have this cosmetic blight called vitiligo, be assured that it is not a sign of cancer.

While this pigmentary failure can occur in all races, the cosmetic—as well as the psychological—implications are considerably greater for those with darker skins. Vitiligo is a dramatic process in dark-skinned people, often causing profound despair. In India, for example, vitiligo is considered by the populace to be a sign of leprosy. Nehru, realizing the myths and superstitions surrounding this perfectly benign condition, felt a treatment for vitiligo was as important for his people as the treatment for leprosy and tuberculosis.

Vitiligo is usually a progressive and relentless disease. Rarely do people with the condition regain their color spontaneously. There may be a long period of time where the depigmented patches remain unchanged, and very often an emotional upset, infection, or illness may activate the process again. The old spots get larger and new spots develop.

Unfortunately, there is no reliable method of regaining lost pigment. Current therapy consists of taking a special pill (a psoralen) and exposing the affected skin to sunlight or long-wave ultraviolet radiation (UVA). This form of therapy—commonly called the PUVA treatment (from **P**soralen **U**ltra**V**iolet **A**)—is similar to the way dermatologists treat extensive psoriasis. But even this procedure may have to be carried out for a number of months or years before any noticeable repigmentation occurs.

Not everyone is a good candidate for repigmentation. Ideally, the person should meet the following criteria:

- The candidate should be in good health. Pregnant women should not be treated.
- For people over twenty years of age, pigment loss should be less than five years.
- The candidate should be at least ten years old.
- Because treatment is a long process, the person must be committed to it and have the time to follow through.

There are some physicians—I am one of them—who treat vitiligo with small doses of anti-inflammatory drugs such as aspirin or ibuprofen along with antibiotics (on the basis that some minor, hidden infection is causing some defect in the immune system). But before you embark on such a regimen, you should ask your general doctor or dermatologist about possible adverse side effects.

Some dermatologists have been using a "cocktail" of the following over-the-counter supplements along with directions for use, and have reported "good results":

Day 1: Vitamin E—600 I.U.

Day 2: Methionine—500 milligrams

Day 3: Selenium—200 mcg

Repeat this cycle for a "long period." And be patient!

The prognosis for vitiligo is discouraging at best. Whatever the treatment, only about one in five patients respond at all, and relapses are the rule. When the involved loss of pigment is in small patches, certain types of makeup (such as Covermark or Dermablend) and concealers can help camouflage the patches of vitiligo.

For more information concerning vitiligo, write to:
National Vitiligo Foundation
P.O. Box 6337, Tyler, Texas 75711
903-534-2925
or www.aad.org
1-888-462-DERM x22

Recap

- All of us—black, yellow, red, and white people—have the same number of melanocytes—special pigment cells—in our skin.
- The most common cause of excessive pigmentation is an increased stimulation in the production of melanin due to certain hormonal changes, sun exposure, or a combination of both.
- Melasma is especially common in young white women, who often develop this blotchiness on their foreheads, cheeks, and mustache areas. It occurs frequently during pregnancy, in women taking oral contraceptives, and is more common in brunettes than in blonds.
- Vitiligo is a mysterious malady characterized by a gradual or rapid loss of pigment, or skin color. If affects about one out of every hundred people and is more common among younger individuals.

9 Sun-Related Skin Conditions

The suntan. The envy of friends and relatives. The golden, tawny bodies on the sand. The bronzed lifeguard. The sad truth is that sun tanning is a dangerous habit with no benefit except the elusive psychological one: looking good and healthy means feeling good and healthy. Exposure to the sun is directly and ultimately responsible for the leathery look of prematurely aged skin, wrinkles, and skin cancer—all of which are irreversible. It can also cause sun poisoning.

The serious problems caused by the sun's rays are getting worse as a result of the thinning of the ozone layer in the earth's atmosphere. The ozone layer normally gives us some protection from the sun, but due to aerosols, propellants, nitrogen oxides from nuclear explosions and supersonic transports, and chlorine from space shuttles, this protective layer has virtually disappeared.

The sun produces several kinds of rays. Two of the rays (Ultraviolet A—UVA and Ultraviolet B—UVB) cause most of the damage to the skin. No ultraviolet rays are safe! (There is also an Ultraviolet C ray—found in fluorescent and germicidal lamps, and Infra Red rays—emitted by light bulbs, heat lamps, space heaters, stoves and furnaces—but these rays do not play a role in the information that follows.)

The sun's harmful rays are more intense in our summer, at high altitudes and the closer you are to the Equator. These harmful effects are increased by reflections from water, snow, sand and cement.

197

The following chapters describe the process behind sun-tanning, how to suntan properly, and how to treat and prevent sun-poisoning.

SUN TANNING

Tanning is nothing more than the efficient, protective mechanism of the body: a response to injury from sunlight and a way to protect us from additional injury. That "healthy-looking" tan, usually associated with good health and enviable sex appeal, is, in fact, damaged skin. The best suntan is no suntan at all!

In early times, sun-tanned skin was associated with those who worked outdoors for a living—the peasants, the farmers, the serfs. People of means, those from the upper social classes and nobility, took pains to stay out of the sun to preserve their natural color. Medieval beauties were admired for their indoor pallor, while the traditional fresh fairness of Englishwomen, a combination of genes, high humidity, and minimum sunlight, has been extolled by lovers and envied by other women.

Because the tanning mechanism is not 100 percent efficient, repeated sun exposure allows certain wavelengths of light to penetrate this defense barrier, causing various sun-related skin conditions.

The more subtle changes caused by the sun's rays may not be apparent for decades, but they do and will occur in every person who is foolish enough to expose himself or herself to excess. Therefore, the only good suntan is no suntan at all.

Compare the sun-exposed portions of your body—your face, hands, forearms—with those parts of your anatomy (your buttocks, for example) that are almost never exposed. Note the difference in smoothness and texture. Your buttocks are young; your hands and face are old. (Everyone should look at his or her buttocks in the mirror and think: This is how my face should look!)

For you fair-haired, fair-skinned, and blue-eyed people, tanning, if it does occur, is a slow process. You have much smaller pigment cells than your dark-haired, darker-skinned, brown-eyed neighbors. So you burn more easily and require infinitely more sun exposure to produce even a modest tan. If you are dark-skinned, on the other hand, merely a brief exposure to the sun often produces a lasting tan.

198

For you light-skinned people who, despite all admonition, still desire that bronzed look, here are a few rules:

- *Acquire your tan gradually.* If you head for the beaches, the backyards, and the lake in order to soak up that first Sunday sun in June, avoid a severe and painful sunburn by limiting your first exposure to fifteen or twenty minutes. Increase the exposure gradually by twenty or thirty minutes a day for four or five more days. The first pigment cells will then begin to show up to darken and protect the skin. From then on, you can tolerate almost any length of exposure.
- If you are a redhead or a blond, you do not have adequate pigment cells to begin with; therefore, you must be more careful and reduce the early exposure times by approximately half.

All this, however, is trial and error. Only *you* will know how much sun you can tolerate on first and subsequent exposures without causing painful sunburn.

- Keep in mind that the most intense rays of the sun occur between 10 AM and 2 PM (standard time), the overhead sun being the strongest. You cannot get sunburned before 9 AM and after 5 PM, at which times the sharply angulated "burn" rays have been filtered out by the atmosphere.
- Also, do not let overcast skies fool you: sunburn can occur on hazy and foggy days. And don't think that only direct exposure to the sun produces burning or tanning. Reflected rays from sand, cement, and water can also cause severe sunburn. Beach umbrellas do not offer absolute protection. And you can even get sunburned while swimming under water!
- *Use suntan creams and lotions.* Many of the suntan preparations—creams, lotions, ointments, gels, sticks, lip balms, etc.—contain specific chemicals that either block out or selectively absorb the shorter wavelengths of sunlight responsible for burning. This may permit some of the longer wavelengths of light—the tanning rays—to penetrate the skin. Sunscreens should be applied about 30 minutes before going outdoors.

People are classified into various skin types depending on their levels of melanin pigmentation. The simplest classification—the one I prefer—is as follows:

- *Skin Type I:* People with fair hair and fair skin or freckles are most susceptible to the rays of the sun. They can develop severe sunburn in a matter of minutes and also have a higher risk of developing skin cancers and wrinkles. If you are Skin Type I, you will not tan no matter how long you bake in the sun. Persistent sunbathing is not only futile, but also downright dangerous.
- *Skin Type II:* These people are also fair-skinned but not as sensitive to the sun's rays as those of Type I. They usually burn and only occasionally develop a "weak" tan.
- *Skin Type III:* This type includes people with darker skin who usually tan but sometimes burn.
- *Skin Type IV:* These people always tan well and almost never develop sunburn.

Depending upon the type of skin you have, there is a wide range of sunscreen products that are rated according to the degree of protection they can give against ultraviolet radiation. This rating is called the Sun Protection Factor (SPF).

This SPF is a guide and a numbering system to assess the efficacy of sunscreen agents. The number represents the number of times longer you can stay in the sun if you use the product than if you used nothing. A number 15 sunscreen, for example, will provide 15 times the user's natural skin protection. In other words, let us say you are susceptible to developing mild sunburn after being out in the sun for one hour. If you apply an SPF-15 sunscreen before sunbathing, you will be able to lie out in the sun for 15 hours before developing your mild burn. (Who is going to lie out in the sun for 15 hours at a stretch?) And you will see all kinds of SPF numbers ranging from 2 to 50!

I believe *everyone*—every skin type—should use an SPF-15 sunscreen. As far as I am concerned, the numbers higher than 15 are meaningless. An SPF-15 sunscreen will filter out 93 percent of the harmful UVB rays. Isn't that enough for most individuals?

When using any sun-protection product, follow the directions given by the manufacturer, and reapply it every two or three hours. Always reapply after swimming.

The best approach to sun-tanning is common sense. This large envelope we call the skin has to last a lifetime, so give it the protection it deserves.

A word about the tanning salons that have sprung up all over the country. Although using the "safer" long-wave ultraviolet rays (UVA), the lamps used in these salons are fraught with the same hazards as other forms of radiation. There are definite dangers associated with repeated exposure to UVA. These rays go deeper into the skin and, in addition to the premature aging, wrinkles, the loss of elasticity, and the potential for developing skin cancer, other harmful effects may include:

- Damage to the eyes, resulting in cataracts.
- Aggravation of existing skin damage caused by sun exposure.
- Aggravation of "light-sensitive" skin disorders, such as cold sores and lupus erythematosus.
- Damage to older people who already have thinner skin.
- Adverse allergic reactions to certain soaps, toiletries, high blood pressure medications, tranquilizers, medications for diabetes, birth control pills, etc.
- Damage to the immune system making the body more susceptible to cancers and infections.
- Damage to the vascular system.

In addition, there are many reported cases of people "catching" lice, scabies, herpes, fungous infections, warts, tinea versicolor, and other infectious diseases from those salons that are not strict about sanitizing their equipment.

One famous dermatologist once said, "I could never understand why people would pay to get skin cancer when they can get it free!"

Do your skin—and yourself—a favor: stay away from those artificial tanning rays.

Children's Skin

Since children often spend hours playing in the sun, protecting children's skin from the sun's harmful rays is one of the most important ways to promote their long-term health. Before sun exposure, always apply a sunscreen with an SPF of at least 15 to any child's skin over the age of six months. Sun protection in childhood is extremely important to prevent skin cancer later in life.

SUN POISONING

Sun poisoning is a nonscientific term that refers to a variety of sun-allergic responses. Light-skinned people, who have less protective skin pigment, are especially susceptible to sun poisoning, but it can occur in anyone who is exposed to enough light. It often occurs in combination with a variety of drugs, chemicals, cosmetics, and plants.

The classic example of sun poisoning is sunburn. We all know that redheads suffer more from the effects of the sun's rays than the rest of the population. This is because they lack one of the main defense mechanisms against sunburn, sufficient melanin pigment in the skin. Black people rarely suffer from sunburn because the pigment in their epidermis (the upper layers of the skin) prevents the penetration of the sunburn rays to the sensitive, deeper layers of the skin.

If you are a susceptible person, certain common drugs can change your normal protective response to the sun. The result can be a severe rash with blisters from the slightest exposure to sunlight or even fluorescent lighting.

Drugs most commonly involved in this type of reaction are the sulfa drugs, "relatives" of tetracycline, various tranquilizers, high blood pressure medication, birth control pills, and oral medications used for diabetes and fungous infections (ringworm).

Direct contact with certain chemicals followed by sun exposure also can cause sun poisoning. The most common substances that cause these "sun-allergic" responses are found in deodorant bar soaps, detergents, certain suntan lotions, shampoos, "first-aid" creams, and various cosmetics and toiletries.

Chemicals found in a variety of vegetables and fruits can cause sun-sensitive reactions. Gardeners and farmers who spend time in the sun and handle such foods as carrots, celery, parsnips, figs, and limes are especially susceptible. Sun poisoning has also been reported as a result of using herbal shampoos followed by sun exposure.

The symptoms of sun allergy are severe itching and rash that occur a few days after the combination of the chemical substance and the light. This sensitivity can be so pronounced that a minute amount of the substance left on your skin followed by exposure to even fluorescent light, may trigger a reaction.

The treatment for sun poisoning is essentially the same as for any allergic dermatitis, such as poison ivy dermatitis. If your case is mild, use wet compresses or soothing baths followed by calamine lotion to relieve your symptoms. If your itching is more persistent, take an antihistamine. For any severe reaction accompanied by intense itching and blisters that weep and ooze, see your dermatologist. You may need treatment for dehydration and possible infection.

PREVENTING SUN POISONING

Preventing sun-sensitive reactions may take a lot of trial and error to determine which drug, chemical, or plant is the culprit. Once you have discovered it, eliminate it from your routine. If the offender is a drug essential to your health (high blood pressure pills or antidiabetic medications for example), you will need to stay out of the sun at all times.

If you are fair-skinned, the best way to avoid a sun-sensitive reaction is to avoid the sun. If this is just not possible, then tan slowly and cautiously.

To prevent overexposure to the sun, use a good sunscreen. Sunscreens usually contain chemicals that selectively block out or absorb all the harmful "short" ultraviolet rays, permitting some of the longer, tanning rays to get through to the skin.

A good but cosmetically inelegant sun-blocking preparation is plain zinc oxide ointment.

To protect the delicate areas of the lips, use a lip balm that contains a sun-blocking agent.

And, finally, before you go out in the sun, remember to:
Slip, Slap, and **Slop!**
Slip on a shirt; **Slap** on a hat; and **Slop** on sunscreen!

For further information on sun-related problems, log on to:
www.aad.org
1-888-462-DERM

Recap

- Tanning is nothing more than the efficient, protective mechanism of the body: a response to injury from sunlight and a way to protect us from additional injury.
- The SPF is a guide and a numbering system to assess the efficacy of sunscreen agents. The number represents how many times longer you can stay in the sun if you use the product than if you used nothing.
- A note about children's skin: since children often spend many hours playing in the sun, protecting children's skin from the sun's harmful rays is one of the most important ways to promote their long-term health.
- There are many reported cases of people "catching" lice, scabies, herpes, fungous infections, warts, tinea versicolor, and other infectious diseases from certain tanning salons that are not strict about sanitizing their tanning equipment.

10
Sports-Related Skin Problems

SKIN PROBLEMS FOR ATHLETES

All of us Americans seem to have at least one favorite **sports** activity—jogging, cycling, tennis, swimming, skiing, backpacking, mountain climbing—you name it. With so many active people, it's not surprising that there are frequent injuries and illnesses related to sports.

As healthy as exercise is, certain hazards go along with it, including the increased possibility of injury to your skin. You also expose yourself to contagious skin diseases in the locker room, on gym mats, and from direct contact with infected people. And, finally, from the sweating, friction and stress you may put yourself through, you create the ideal environment for new skin conditions to develop or for existing ones to get worse.

From acne to sun poisoning, from herpes to *"jogger's nipples,"* from *"turf toe"* to *"bikini bottom,"* the competitive and weekend athlete alike risk a litany of skin problems. But you can prevent or lessen them with proper care.

Let's look at some of these sports-related skin troubles. You'll find many of these conditions described in other chapters of this book.

Boxing, Wrestling and Other Close Contact Sports

Anytime you have close contact with another person, you

expose yourself to possible bacterial and viral infections. One common hazard of close contact sports is *impetigo*, a highly contagious bacterial infection you can get from infected opponents as well as from dirty gym mats. Impetigo gets a foothold on damaged skin, a common result of the friction and scraping from wrestling and other contact sports.

Boils are bacterial infections of the hair follicle. These painful, shiny, bright-red swellings of the skin usually develop over the elbows, forearms and knees after a bruise or break in the skin. You should see a physician if you think you have boils.

Herpes simplex infections and *dimple warts* are viral infections frequently associated with contact sports. Herpes simplex infections are so common in wrestlers that they're sometimes called "herpes gladiatorum." The highly contagious dimple warts (molluscum contagiosum) also plague wrestlers, spreading easily in the warm, moist areas caused by heavy sweat.

And, if infections aren't enough, close contact sports also increase the risk of *scabies*, a very contagious and terribly itchy infestation. Scabies mites can live on dirty gym mats and on the bodies of your opponents.

Finally, close contact sports encourage a variety of other attacks on your skin including *cuts, bruises, lacerations, abrasions* and *mat burns*.

Football, Baseball, Hockey and Other Team Sports

Some team sports create special problems because of the combination of rough activity and tight-fitting, bulky padding and uniforms.

"Acne mechanica," an infection of hair follicles where the concentration of oil glands is high, results from the rubbing, pressure, heat and sweating caused by bulky sports equipment, football helmets, catcher's masks, and heavy protective padding. Also by performing bench presses.

Boils are another common problem because of frequent skin injuries and the warm, moist conditions these infections love to grow in.

206

Turf toe and *turf burns* are unique skin problems caused by playing on artificial turf. Turf toe appears as red, swollen and painful big toes that result from playing alternately on natural and artificial surfaces. Turf burns are abrasions that scrape off part of the skin, usually over the elbows, forearms and knees.

Swimming and Other Water Sports

Long distance swimmers often suffer from a bacterial infection called *swimmer's ear*. Exposure to water for a long time dissolves the normal oils in the ear canals, softening and weakening the tissues. Unfriendly bacteria can multiply and cause itching, swelling, pain, tenderness and a yellowish discharge from the ear. *Dimple warts* are also a common problem in swimmers.

Seabather's eruption, also known as "sea lice," is a distinctive itchy rash that is caused by the "thimble jellyfish," an organism that thrives in marine waters off Florida, in the Gulf of Mexico and the Caribbean. The characteristic symptom of this hypersensitivity reaction is that the rash and itching occur underneath swimsuits and T-shirts—on the non-exposed portions of the body as opposed to *swimmer's itch*, that attacks the exposed areas of the body. *Swimmer's itch* is caused by the larvae of a parasite (a schistosome) that enters the pores of the skin when the swimmer leaves the water. As the water droplets evaporate from the skin, and the swimmer dries off, these worm-like larvae burrow under the skin causing an unpleasant, itchy rash.

"Bikini bottom" is a mild infection of the skin that results from wearing a wet bathing suit. This annoying infection frequently shows up when the sweat pores become clogged, trapping the bacteria that usually live on the skin in friendly and harmless numbers. Unable to escape, the trapped germs begin to proliferate, spread and cause trouble.

Green hair: Blonds who swim a lot in pools may find that their hair has turned green! This startling color change is due to copper additives used in swimming pools. Peroxide bleaching solutions will return the hair to its normal color.

Running and Jogging

A common problem for runners and joggers are *plantar warts*, warts on the soles of the feet. The warm, moist habitat of running shoes encourages the growth of the virus that causes these warts. *Corns* are another problem of joggers. These are often caused by improperly fitting shoes, especially those that are too narrow.

"*Jogger's toe*," also known as "*tennis toe*," is a complaint of joggers, runners, tennis players and mountain climbers. Appearing as a bruise beneath the toenails, usually on the big toes, this harmless discoloration is caused by ill-fitting shoes and sudden stops which force the toes into the front of the shoe, bending the nails and breaking the blood vessels. Soft, comfortable shoes with plenty of room and trimming the toenail straight across, can prevent this problem of "short stops."

"*Jogger's nipples*" is an uncomfortable problem that can affect both sexes. It's an injury caused by friction in women who run without wearing bras and in men who jog in cotton T- shirts. The nipples become sore and red and may even bleed. To prevent this annoying condition, coat your nipples with Vaseline and wear a bra or shirt with a smooth, hard finish, such as those made of silk or semi-synthetic fabrics.

Gymnastics, Aerobics and Dancing

Gymnasts, dancers and others who do heavy stretching activity commonly develop *stretch marks*. These are thin scars that show up when the skin is distended or stretched over a long period of time. They are *not* a sign of disease.

Gymnasts may also suffer from *warts* on their palms and fingers. This common viral infection can spread from contact with gym mats, parallel bars and other gymnastics equipment.

Outdoor Sports

Direct exposure to the sun or rays reflected off snow, sand and water can create skin problems for both summer and winter athletes. *Sunburn* and *sun poisoning* are common in baseball and tennis players, golfers, mountain climbers, swimmers and skiers. For skiers and mountain climbers, it's important to remember that the effects of ultraviolet light are stronger at higher altitudes. Taking medications, such as antibiotics or tranquilizers, may increase your risk of sunburn or sun poisoning. To prevent sun-related skin problems year round, always apply protective sunscreens before you go out in the sun.

Warm weather athletes are often pestered by *insect bites* and *stings*. Make sure to pack a good, protective insect repellent in your sports bag—and use it!

Winter sports carry the added risk of *frostbite* from exposure to extreme cold. Wearing several layers of thin clothing, rather than one or two heavier layers, can help prevent frostbite. Also, because natural skin oil offers some protection to the skin, wait to shave and wash your face *after* you've come in from cold weather.

Skiers frequently suffer from *dry, chapped skin* caused by winter's low temperatures and low relative humidity.

General Sports Activities

Heavy sweating, heat and tight-fitting clothing go along with many sports activities and play a part in softening and weakening the upper layers of the skin that normally protect us against the invasion and spread of harmful microorganisms—bacteria, viruses, fungi, and the scabies mite.

Athlete's foot is the infection most clearly associated with sports. Caused by a fungus, this mildly contagious disorder spreads where there is heavy sweating and poor foot hygiene. It's a frequent visitor in locker rooms, shower stalls and other warm, moist surroundings where bare feet tread (see page 78).

Jock itch is a common infection of the groin caused by a fungus or yeast. Like athlete's foot, it's related to sweating and warm, moist environments (see page 83).

Allergic rashes are troublesome to all types of athletes and can be caused by many natural or manufactured products: plants (poison ivy), clothing (shoes, gloves), and sports equipment (leather grips of racquets and golf clubs, basketballs, barbells, wet suits and rubber diving masks, Fiberglas in hockey sticks, gym mats, adhesive tape, etc.). Sweating always makes these allergic rashes worse.

Heat, perspiration, friction, sun exposure and the emotional stress of competitive sports can cause or aggravate many skin problems. *Acne*, for example, is worsened by the pressure and friction of the face masks, helmets and the bulky padding of football uniforms. *Eczema* flares up with heat, perspiration and emotional stress. *Hives* can be provoked by heavy exercise, quick changes in body temperature, and stress.

In addition, athletic activities expose you to a whole batch of skin injuries. Wearing new or poorly fitting shoes and subjecting your feet to friction and pressure they're not used to can quickly lead to *friction blisters* on your feet and toes. These can be treated by letting your feet rest, keeping them dry, wearing two pairs of socks—each of a different fabric—and using a foot powder.

Slamming your feet down can cause a pinching type of injury called "*black heel*." As its name says, this condition appears as a black patch over the heel caused by small hemorrhages or bleeding in the upper layers of the skin, often causing concern that it might be a malignancy. It occurs almost exclusively in teenagers who play hard surface sports (basketball, tennis, handball and squash) and it disappears without treatment.

Callus formation, particularly on the feet, is the most common mechanical injury in athletes. Calluses, and their close cousins *corns*, are the skin's natural reaction to repeated rubbing and friction. Firm, thickened patches develop at points of pressure, especially over bony spots such as your heels. Gymnasts, oarsmen, golfers and tennis players often develop them on their hands. You can treat calluses by reducing the friction or pressure with pads, wraps or orthopedic appliances.

Ingrown toenails are often found on the big toes of many athletes and result from poorly fitting or tight shoes and poor hygiene.

Even though athletes can always expect injuries, including those to the skin, there's no reason to be fearful about participating in competitive or recreational sports. You can prevent trouble by practicing good hygiene (soap and water!), wearing clothing and sports equipment that fit properly, and protecting yourself from the sun, intense cold, and insects. Remember that the best offense is a good defense. Protect yourself—and your skin.

For further information about sports-related skin problems, log on to:
www.aad.org
1-888-462-DERM x22

Recap

- Any time you have close contact with another person, you expose yourself to possible bacterial and viral infections.
- Heavy sweating, heat and tight-fitting clothing go along with many sports activities and play a part in softening and weakening the upper layers of the skin that normally protect us against the invasion and spread of harmful microorganisms.
- Ingrown toenails are often found on the big toes of many athletes and result from poorly fitting or tight shoes and poor hygiene.

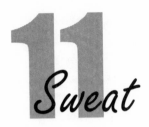

Sweat

"It is not manly to fear sweat."
—Seneca, *Moral Epistles to Lucilius*, XXXI, vii, 31

All normal, healthy people sweat. Some more, some less. And all healthy people smell when they sweat. This, too, is normal.

Sweat is important in regulating your body temperature. Despite enormous changes in the temperature of our external environment—be it tropical or sub-zero—your internal body temperature remains fairly constant.

When you are exposed to excessive heat, the sweat glands pour out their watery secretion (sweat) and carry out the vital task of cooling your body. This thermoregulatory mechanism has allowed us to adapt to the hottest climates.

Sweat is composed of the secretion of two types of glands: the 2 million eccrine glands distributed over the entire body, and the localized apocrine glands, which are restricted primarily to the armpits, the anogenital region, and the nipples. The growth of the apocrine glands is regulated by a hormone that begins to form about the time of puberty and decreases markedly in old age. (This is why children under the age of twelve and elderly people do not suffer from "body odor.") These apocrine glands become active after puberty, respond to hormonal secretions, and are stimulated by emotional factors such as stress and sexual excitement.

Sweat itself is essentially odorless. Most of the odor is due to the action of various bacteria on the milky secretion of the apocrine sweat glands. These bacteria are most active in moist and warm environments, particularly hairy armpits.

Sweat from body regions devoid of apocrine glands can also have an unpleasant odor. For example, the odor of certain aromatic foods and spices (such as garlic and onions) are secreted in eccrine sweat. And eccrine sweat, from prolonged exercising, can cause an unpleasant odor due to bacterial action on the soft, wet skin. This is the most common cause of foot odor.

Normally, we lose about 2 quarts of liquid through perspiration each day. Perspiration is not under voluntary control. You cannot decide when you want to perspire and you cannot tell yourself to stop this mechanism. Emotional and environmental factors (heat) influence the degree of sweating, especially over the palms, soles, armpits, and forehead; and doctors believe that cigarette smoking may also be responsible for excessive perspiration. You can, however, "harness" this mechanism somewhat by using antiperspirants and deodorants.

Antiperspirants are compounds that reduce the volume of perspiration. Deodorants are products used to mask, diminish, or prevent perspiration odor.

Antiperspirants

Antiperspirants are sold as pads, creams, sprays, lotions, powders, liquids, and roll-ons. We don't know for certain how antiperspirants act, but we believe that they reduce perspiration by strictly mechanical means. Made up almost exclusively of aluminum salts, they act by either shrinking the pores, blocking the openings of the pores, or causing the sweat to be reabsorbed below the skin's surface.

No antiperspirant completely stops the flow of perspiration. And since the secretion of sweat is an essential function of the skin for temperature regulation and water metabolism, it would not be desirable if it did.

Antiperspirants should be used daily, as it takes two weeks to build up maximum protection. For best results, apply to clean skin, but not immediately after shaving. Roll-ons and creams usually give greater protection than aerosols, but the choice of one type over another is a matter of personal preference: ease of application, lack of messiness, the absence of burning or stinging, and which TV commercial appeals to you. In cases of excessive perspiration (known as diaphoresis or hyperhidrosis), there is a prescription solution called Drysol, which, when used as directed, is remarkably effective in reducing the amount of underarm sweating. An over-the-counter preparation—Certain Dri—has been very successful in many of my patients suffering from excessive perspiration.

Deodorants

Deodorants are available as powders, creams, sticks, pads, roll-ons, soaps, or sprays, and are effective for a few hours to several days. They do not in any way affect the flow of perspiration. Unlike the perfumes, colognes, and toilet waters of a previous era that merely masked perspiration odor, these products use antibacterial agents, such as neomycin, triclosan (found in certain deodorant soaps), and other bacteria-destroying chemicals, to reduce or eliminate the offending bacteria.

Some people are allergic to the popular, commercial deodorant preparations. If so, try any of the (so-called) hypoallergenic products.

Deodorants that do not claim to check perspiration are classified as cosmetics. If the same preparation is labeled an "antiperspirant," it becomes a drug, as it alleges to change a bodily function.

In addition to antiperspirants and deodorants, there are several general measures you can take to prevent body odor:

- Bathe frequently. Nothing beats personal cleanliness for eliminating odors.
- Keep your clothing clean. Clothing collects not only the odors but also the germs responsible for them.
- Wear only cotton shirts and blouses. Polyester fibers do not "breathe," and they often retain odor even after laundering.
- Shave your armpits regularly. Bacteria *love* armpits.
- Avoid garlic, onions, and asparagus. These can produce offensive odors, especially in the summertime.
- Cut down on caffeine (coffee, tea, and cola drinks) which stim-

ulates sweat gland activity.

- For excessive perspiration and perspiration odor of the feet, try the "tea-bag remedy" described on page 249.

One of the latest methods of how to rid yourself of excess sweating is by the injection of Botox—botulinum toxin—into the affected areas. Still in the experimental stages, this has worked in a number of patients in people with severe sweaty armpits.

Is it difficult to get rid of perspiration odor? No sweat!

For further information about sweat, log on to: www.aad.org
1-888-462-DERM x22
or for Certain Dri, contact
www.numarklabs.com/products/otc/

Recap

- Sweat is important in regulating your body temperature. Despite enormous changes in the temperature of our external environment—be it tropical or sub-zero—your internal body temperature remains fairly constant.
- Antiperspirants are compounds that reduce the volume of perspiration. Deodorants are products used to mask, diminish, or prevent perspiration odor.
- No antiperspirant completely stops the flow of perspiration. And since the secretion of sweat is an essential function of the skin for temperature regulation and water metabolism, it would not be desirable if it did.
- Deodorants that do not claim to check perspiration are classified as cosmetics. If the same preparation is labeled an "antiperspirant," it becomes a drug, as it alleges to change a bodily function.

For further information about sweating, log on to: www.aad.org
or http://www.numarklabs.com/products/otc/
1-888-462-DERM x22

12 The Skin of Your Feet

When we gaze into a mirror, what usually gets most of our attention? I'll tell you. Our face, our eyes, our hair, and our figure. We almost never look down at those faraway appendages called feet. Because, like Alice in Wonderland growing taller while eating her cake, we say to our feet: "I'm too far away to trouble myself about you; and you must manage the best way you can." So most of us never give our feet a second thought—unless they itch, burn, or hurt.

Our foot is actually an intricate structure designed for strength and flexibility. Each foot contains 28 bones, 107 ligaments, 33 joints, and 20 muscles. With each step, an entire network of muscles, bones, and tissues—from toe to calf—goes to work to get our body moving. And moving it does: the average person will walk about 120,000 miles in his or her lifetime—more than four times the circumference of the earth.

Our feet suffer harsher treatment than any other portion of our anatomy. They bear the weight of our body, pound the pavement, and spend most of our waking hours stuffed into dark, tight shoes. And although they take decades of punishing service, our feet serve us admirably; they propel us through life, providing balance, support, and motion.

Encasing this highly capable, sensitive marvel of design is the skin of the foot. Different from the skin on any other part of the body, the sole of the foot is fifteen times thicker than the skin of the face and three times thicker than the skin of the palm.

While we trap our feet all day in shoes that don't permit them to "breathe," the 250,000 sweat glands continue to pour out about a half pint of perspiration every day. Inside a pair of shoes, feet swelter in a tropical environment with 80-degree heat and 80 percent humidity, making an ideal breeding ground for microorganisms: bacteria, viruses, and fungi. (The toewebs possess 1,000 times the number of bacteria that can be found on other portions of the skin.)

As we get older, our feet begin to lose their natural resilience; heel pain is common because the fat padding of the sole begins to wear thin; and the skin of the feet becomes thinner and loses some of its elasticity. Proper foot care for the elderly is essential: healthy feet allow older people the opportunity to remain physically active and independent.

Basic Foot Care For Comfort & Beauty

A beautiful foot—and there are beautiful feet—is one that feels supple, exhibits soft heels, has smooth toenails, has no odor, and displays no corns or calluses.

Here is how to make the skin of our feet look and feel great:

- Use good daily hygiene. That means washing your feet daily using an antibacterial soap.
- Always dry your feet and toewebs thoroughly.
- Use a medicated foot powder.
- Wear cotton socks, if possible.
- Wear shoes that fit.
- Soak feet for 20 to 30 minutes at the end of the day in warm water using special bath crystals.
- After drying, massage your feet with a foot cream.
- Trim toenails straight across to prevent ingrown nails.
- Treat your feet to an occasional pedicure.

SKIN CONDITIONS OF THE FEET

Dry Skin

Even though feet perspire and lose about half a pint of fluid each day, the moisture released from the sweat glands can evaporate quickly. Environmental factors, such as low relative humidity and extremes of heat and cold can dry out the skin, as can frequent bathing with harsh soaps. When moisture is lost, the outer, protective layer of the skin loses its flexibility and becomes dry and brittle. About seven out of ten adult women complain of rough, dry skin on their feet and legs, a phenomenon that is more common in the wintertime.

To prevent dry skin of the feet, pamper them regularly. After a long day, soak your feet in warm water for about 30 minutes to soothe and re-moisturize them. Adding bath crystals made especially for the feet will help soften not only the upper layers of the skin but any corns and calluses you may have. After soaking, pat your feet dry with a soft towel and remove any dry, flaky residue with a pumice stone or callus file. Then gently massage a moisturizing cream specifically designed to penetrate the thick skin of the sole, which will enhance the skin's ability to absorb moisture. And do not sleep under electric blankets.

Cracked Heels

More than 18 million adults—and one in every seven women—suffer from cracked, painful heels. This is a result of excessively dry skin, the heels being especially susceptible to cracking because there are continually subjected to friction and pressure.

To relieve painful cracked heels, soak your feet for 30 minutes in a moisturizing bath as described above, pat dry, and then apply a soothing, emollient foot cream to soften the heels, allay the pain and help prevent infection. There is a very helpful prescription product—Lac-Hydrin Cream—that, when applied once or twice daily after a bath, will help relieve all the symptoms of dry heels.

Athlete's Foot

Athlete's foot is discussed on page 78.

Warts

Warts are discussed on page 28.

CORNS AND CALLUSES

Corns and calluses are common foot problems. Characterized by layers of compacted dead skin cells, these protective mechanisms of the skin develop as a result of abnormal, prolonged friction and pressure between the shoe—often a tight or ill-fitting one—and the skin.

Corns

Beginning as red, irritated skin over an underlying bony prominence, these painful and unsightly, cone-shaped areas of thickened skin are among the most common ailments to which the human foot is subject. Pressure of these hard, conical masses on sensitive nerve endings causes the pain and tenderness.

Depending upon where the corn is located, it is either hard or soft. In general, corns on the top of the toes are hard; those between the toes are soft.

Hard corns are indicative of concentrated pressure over the toes and sole of the foot, the result of deformity or dysfunction of the foot or toes. The hard, central core of these corns is often embedded in surrounding callus.

Soft corns form between the toes, almost exclusively in the fourth web space (the last toeweb), as a result of pressure of the joint of one toe pressing against the other. The characteristic softness of these growths is due to the retention of moisture; mainly sweat, which, as a result of the close proximity of the toes, is unable to evaporate.

Treating Corns

The first step in eliminating hard corns is to remove the cause of rubbing and friction. Wear properly fitting shoes or stretch the toe of the shoe; for immediate relief, cut off that portion of the shoe at the point where the pressure is greatest.

At the first sign of redness, use moleskin to provide protection for the affected areas. Soak feet in a footbath with special footbath crystals, use a corn file to remove the rough, dry skin and apply corn remover pads to ease the painful pressure.

To treat—and prevent—soft corns, keep the toewebs separated

with lamb's wool or one-inch squares of cotton material (not, however, cotton balls or batting) at all times, and dust on a foot powder. By reducing the pressure that was responsible for the corn in the first place, these growths usually disappear by themselves.

Calluses

A callus is a thickened mass of skin that can form on any portion of the body. Like corns, calluses develop to protect sensitive skin from continued friction and pressure.

Calluses on the hands are very common and often indicate the type of work one does. Calluses on the bottom and sides of the feet arise where weight-bearing pressures of the body are concentrated. These calluses are hard, dry, horny-like masses of yellowish skin. Unlike corns, they do not have a central core. As the calloused skin thickens and hardens, it begins to press on sensitive nerve endings, causing pain and discomfort.

Treating Calluses

The solution to the treatment and prevention of calluses of the feet is simple: wear shoes that fit properly. Shoes should be wide enough so that the foot can expand to its full width.

Redistributing the weight evenly over the entire ball of the foot using cushioned pads made of felt or foam rubber is a popular method used in relieving and preventing callus formation.

For the long-standing calluses, there are special foot bath soaks, callus files, callus cushions and removers, and other products especially designed for these thickened and oftentimes painful masses.

For further information about foot problems, log on to
www.aad.org
1-888-462-DERM x22

Recap

- Each foot contains 28 bones, 107 ligaments, 33 joints, and 20 muscles.

- Our feet suffer harsher treatment than any other portion of our anatomy: they bear the weight of our body, pound the pavement, and they spend most of our waking hours stuffed into dark, tight shoes.
- As we get older, our feet begin to lose their natural resilience; heel pain is common because the fat padding of the sole begins to wear thin; and the skin of the feet becomes thinner and loses some of its elasticity.

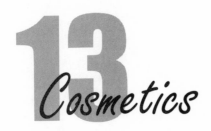

Cosmetics

How you look influences how you feel—physically and emotionally. Physical beauty has always played a significant role in the way people have valued themselves and in the way others have valued them. We are programmed to believe that what is beautiful is also good and true. As a result, those who look neat, well groomed, and appealing to the eye are usually more socially successful and happier than those who do not.

The use of cosmetics is one of the most common methods of achieving a particular image. Put simply, a cosmetic is "an article to be rubbed in, poured, sprinkled, sprayed on, introduced into, or otherwise applied to the human body or any part thereof for cleansing, beautifying, promoting attractiveness or altering the appearance."

The use of cosmetics to adorn our skin and enhance our appearance goes back to the beginning of time. Skillfully used, cosmetics can change your appearance by adding color, texture, form, and shine. They can add a healthy glow to disguise winter pallor and ashiness. They can camouflage minor blemishes and defects. For many women, cosmetics also help build self-confidence and self-esteem.

Cosmetic products, formerly used by only the wealthy, are now available to everyone. What cosmetics you should use is easy: whatever you like, whatever you can afford, and whatever doesn't cause any adverse reactions or side effects as itchiness, oiliness, or pimples. If you like the look, the feel, the smell, and the price—use it!

There are some general guidelines, however, to help you be a better cosmetics consumer:

- The most expensive cosmetic is not necessarily the best for you. What you pay for when you buy expensive cosmetics is fragrance, the designer's name, the cost of advertising, and fancy packaging. The expensive products, however, often have greater esthetic and psychological advantage for the buyer who feels that the more costly the better. It is more chic and statusy, it stresses exclusivity, it has more snob appeal, and it gives the buyer a feeling of well-being. But remember: the active and useful ingredients in all cosmetics are relatively inexpensive and pretty much the same.

- Don't be sucked in by the hype that a cosmetic is "pH-balanced," "dermatologist-tested," and "hypo-allergenic." They all are! And as far as "natural" and "organic," these are meaningless terms intended to impress and confuse you.

- There are no so-called moisturizers or creams that can restore elasticity to damaged skin. And they do not slow down aging. Most moisturizers cause blackheads and whiteheads!

- The best cosmetics are those that are oil-free and water-based.

COSMETIC SAFETY

If used and stored properly, almost all cosmetics—except mascara that has a "life expectancy" of only 3 or 4 months—can last for about one year. Old cosmetics are risky to use and will never give you the proper results. Homemade cosmetics present problems with bacterial contamination.

If your makeup has changed color or odor, dried out, or separated, get rid of it—chances are it's contaminated or has outlived its usefulness.

Cosmetic Do's

- Before you purchase an expensive cosmetic, ask for a sample to try at home.

- Keep the lids and caps of jars, bottles, and tubes tightly closed when not in use.
- Keep your jars, bottles, and tubes scrupulously clean, and store them in well-ventilated places away from excessive heat and cold.
- Clean all your sponges and cosmetic brushes frequently with a mild soap and water.
- Keep your eye pencils clean and freshen them up periodically by sharpening them.
- Change your powder puffs often.
- Always remove your makeup before going to bed.
- To remove your cosmetics, use a tried-and-true product called Albolene.
- Check the expiration date on mascara and other cosmetics.
- Discard your mascara after 3 or 4 months or earlier, if the odor or color has changed. Mascara has a much higher risk of bacterial contamination than other cosmetics. After using mascara, always wipe the brush off with a clean, dry facial tissue.
- If you have a skin or eye infection, your cosmetics can easily become contaminated. Discard any you may have been using, and don't use any cosmetics until your problem has cleared up.

Cosmetic Don'ts

- Never use anyone else's cosmetics and never lend yours to anyone. Swapping cosmetics can lead to contamination and spread infection.
- Never use those so-called "tester" cosmetics from the cosmetic counters. Tester lipsticks can spread the herpes virus, and other tester products can spread infection to the skin and eyes.
- Never put makeup on an unwashed face. Use a mild, gentle soap before applying any cosmetic. And do not use deodorant soaps on your face; they leave an irritating residue on the skin.
- Don't put makeup on first thing in the morning. Let the puffiness of your face disappear first.
- Never apply any eye makeup while in a moving vehicle.
- If you wear contact lenses, don't use mascara with fibers.
- Never add anything to your cosmetics. Water and other liquids encourage bacterial growth.

225

- Avoid cosmetics that contain fragrances.
- And never use any cosmetic that has vitamin E in it! It can only cause allergic rashes on your skin.

A NOTE ON EAR-PIERCING

'Ear ye! 'Ear ye! Piercings are in vogue and teenagers, as well as adults, are having it done.

And one of the latest fads—eerie, in a way—is that some young women are having each ear pierced in three or four different places and wear as many as six or eight earrings at one time. Now belly buttons, nipples, noses, lips, and—yes—tongues!

It may come as a surprise to many, but pierced earrings were common ornaments of men in England up to the seventeenth century! And it was common in the U.S. Navy up to about ninety years ago.

Yet, harmless as the custom may seem, it isn't something that should be done casually by friends, relatives, or other unskilled individuals. The ear-piercing procedure itself takes only a few moments and is relatively painless, but is best performed by a physician with a proper sterile technique and knowledge about the minor hazards that accompany it.

People with certain diseases, such as eczema, rheumatic fever, certain blood disorders, impetigo, the cystic type of acne, and allergies to metals, should not have their ears pierced.

The American Medical Association has warned the public of the complications of ear-piercing, particularly when done under nonsterile conditions. These include hepatitis and other internal infections, in rare cases leading to death; excessive bleeding which may form a blood tumor; raised scars (keloids), which can occur in susceptible people; and allergies to the metal (usually nickel) in the earrings.

Nickel is a powerful sensitizer, especially in contact with broken skin. Almost all earrings contain nickel. Many people believe that their 14-carat or 18-carat gold earrings are safe to use in pierced ears. Not so! The 14-carat gold jewelry has 14 parts gold and 10 parts nickel; the 18-carat gold jewelry has 18 parts gold and 6 parts nickel—enough nickel to cause and prolong allergies. As a result, there has been a "rash" of skin allergies on earlobes that resemble infection. For the most part this reaction is merely an inflammation. Occasionally, however, certain bacteria multiply on the raw, broken skin, resulting in a true infection with weeping, oozing, and crusting. If this occurs, you must consult your doctor.

To prevent this type of allergy, purchase trainer earrings made of surgical stainless steel. In addition to being made of stainless steel, these trainer earrings should be the "post" type. I do not recommend hoops or wires until at least three months after the ear-piercing procedure.

Should you have your ears pierced? If you are healthy, plan to have your ears pierced in a sterile manner by a physician, do not have a history of allergies to metals, and if you have no raised scars on your skin, chances are you will have no complications following your ear-piercing.

Here are some other hints to prevent infection:

- After having your ears pierced, wear the same earrings continuously for at least six weeks.
- Gently wash the front and back of your earlobes with soap and water at least twice daily. (Do not use alcohol to clean these areas, as the alcohol may dissolve or in some way react with the glue that cements the ball to the post.)
- Twirl (turn) the earrings several complete revolutions two or three times daily.

Some redness and tenderness is normal after ear-piercing. If you experience any unusual pain, swelling, or discharge, call the physician who did the procedure.

For further information about cosmetics and skin care products,
log on to: www.aad.org
1-888-462-DERM x22

Recap

- A cosmetic is "an article to be rubbed in, poured, sprinkled or sprayed on, introduced into, or otherwise applied to the human body or any part thereof for cleansing, beautifying, promoting attractiveness or altering the appearance."

- To remove your cosmetics, use a tried-and-true product called Albolene.
- The most expensive cosmetic is not necessarily the best for you. When you buy expensive cosmetics, you pay for fragrance, the designer's name, the cost of advertising, and fancy packaging.
- If used and stored properly, almost all cosmetics—except mascara's "life expectancy" of only 3 or 4 months—can last for about one year.

14
Cosmetic Problems

Cosmetic problems include large pores, various types of scars, keloids, stretch marks, cellulite, the aging skin, and wrinkles.

In the following chapters, I will attempt to define and describe these conditions and disorders, mention some of their causes, and some therapies where possible.

PORES

Show me a person who claims to have the "largest facial pores in the world," and I will show you someone who owns at least one magnifying mirror!

Skin pores are the openings of hair follicles, oil glands, and sweat glands. Because they are inherited, you cannot change their size, no matter what the cosmetic firms tell you.

It is true that certain conditions may make pores "appear" larger or smaller. Oily skin and severe acne, for example, may widen the oil ducts to create the "large pore" appearance. And pores may be more apparent on the nose, cheeks, and chin where there is the greatest concentration of oil glands. Repeated squeezing of blackheads and pimples may also lead to permanently widened pores, some of which may actually be tiny, pitted scars.

Other conditions can make your pores look smaller temporarily. For instance, note what happens to your pores when you sunburn. They become considerably smaller due to the inflammation and swelling around the pores. Once the inflammation has subsided, the pores will return to their original appearance. Pinching or gently slapping the skin of the cheeks to make them pink has a similar, temporary pore-shrinking effect.

There is *no* scientific evidence to support the fact that pores can be made to open and close, as many advertisements would lead you to believe. Certain astringents containing acetone and alcohol, as well as various facial masks, however, can produce a temporary "shrinking" effect. These products help remove excess oil from the skin surface that makes the skin feel cool and tight. A possible explanation of this phenomenon is that the astringent or mask acts as an irritant on the skin surface. This irritation causes swelling around the pore, thus making the opening appear smaller and shrunken. Any shrinkage, however, is so insignificant and so short-lived that the time, effort, and cost involved are usually not worth the outcome.

Similarly, hot baths, hot showers, and hot packs followed by cold baths, cold showers, and cold packs do absolutely nothing to the size of the pores. The only effect of the "hot-cold" theory is the sensation of a tightening, a contraction, a shriveling, whatever in the pores. If, however, it makes you feel good—do it! It cannot do any harm.

For those of you who think your facial pores are the largest, the most ugly, and the most noticeable, do the following:

- Wash your face thoroughly with soap and water three times a day to prevent oils from accumulating, clogging up, and distending the pores.
- Use a good, commercial astringent or facemask that makes you and your skin feel good.
- Use only oil-free and water-based cosmetics and moisturizers.

And throw away your magnifying mirrors…

Recap

- Skin pores are the openings of hair follicles, oil glands, and sweat glands. Because they are inherited, you cannot change their size, no matter what the cosmetic firms tell you.
- Repeated squeezing of blackheads and pimples may also lead to

permanently widened pores, some of which may actually be tiny, pitted scars.

- Hot baths, hot showers, and hot packs followed by cold baths, cold showers, and cold packs do absolutely nothing to the size of the pores.

SCARS

"Though the wound be healed yet the scar remains."
—English Proverb

Almost everyone has at least one scar—from a vaccination, cut or laceration, burn, acne, boil, chicken pox, shingles, or surgical procedures.

Scars come in two varieties—the depressed variety and the raised ones. Some hucksters would have you believe they have "proven" products that will flatten out or eliminate scars. Don't believe them! Massaging scars with creams and potions containing such magical ingredients as turtle oil, placenta extract, cocoa butter, or vitamin E is useless and expensive.

Certain medical procedures, however, can make scars less conspicuous. For the depressed scars, these include dermabrasion (skin planing), treating them with various acids (chemical peels), a type of plastic sheeting (for raised scars), and, for more serious scars, plastic surgery and laser resurfacing treatments.

A relatively new method is being used by dermatologists to treat certain types of depressed scars and defects resulting from scarring diseases such as chicken pox and acne, birth defects, injury, and depressions left after surgery. This procedure is the Zyderm and Zyplast Collagen Implant, and it has been tested in thousands of patients in the past few years.

Collagen is the generic name for a family of proteins that are the major fibrous component of skin, tendons, ligaments, cartilage, and bone. Accounting for about one-third of the total human protein, it acts as the so-called glue of the bodily tissues. (The name is taken from the Greek "kolla," meaning glue.) This jelly-like protein complex is responsible for the smooth, pliable texture of the skin and gives it proper tone, resilience, and elasticity.

In the Zyderm (or Zyplast) Collagen Implant, a physician uses a fine-gauge needle to inject collagen directly into depressed or scarred areas of the skin—those where the original collagen has been lost or destroyed. The implant fills in lines, crags, and depressions, thus raising the skin to the level of surrounding tissues.

Once injected, the implant becomes stationary, and takes on the same texture as normal skin. What is particularly remarkable is that the body accepts this implanted collagen. In fact, it appears that cells and blood vessels actually grow into the implant, making it a living part of the skin.

The number of treatment sessions—and success of the results—will vary with the size, depth, and nature of the depression or scar. Hardened scars may require several injections to soften the tissue, so that subsequent injections can correct it. And occasional "touch-up" implantations may be necessary to maintain the correction.

Adverse reactions to Zyderm are rare. To determine if you are sensitive to the implant material, your dermatologist will administer a test implantation in your forearm. You will be asked to watch the site for four weeks for any signs of sensitivity.

Very deep scars, such as those from severe acne, chicken pox, and other viral infections, do not respond well to the Zyderm Implant. But for many patients this implantation procedure can provide a safer and less expensive alternative to plastic surgery or laser therapy.

For further information about scars, log on to www.aad.org
or phone: 1-888-462-DERM x22

Recap

- Scars come in two varieties—the depressed variety and the raised ones.
- Collagen is the generic name for a family of proteins that make up the major fibrous component of skin, tendons, ligaments, cartilage, and bone. Accounting for about one third of the total human protein, it acts as a sort of glue for the bodily tissues.

KELOIDS

A keloid is an abnormal scar, a bizarre response to injury.

Actually, it is an overgrowth of scar tissue. The scar tissue continues to form long after it is needed, building up extra tissue and resulting in a hard, smooth lump.

Keloids—also known as hypertrophic scars—are a medical mystery. We don't know what causes them. Nor can we predict when, where, in whom they will occur, or how large they'll become. We do know that they are much more common in Asians and blacks, who have a tendency to develop keloids even after minor injuries.

Keloids often develop over earlobes after ear piercing; over the upper arm following vaccinations; over appendectomy and gall bladder operation scars, and over the chest area following acne bumps that have healed. They develop more commonly on the skin of the central portion of the body.

If you have a keloid, don't be alarmed. The only problem it usually causes is cosmetic. In rare instances keloids may be somewhat incapacitating, for example, if they develop across joints.

If the keloid is small and inconspicuous, let it be. For larger lesions and those that are cosmetically unacceptable, your dermatologist can offer a variety of treatments—but no guarantees that they will work. Keloids are highly resistant to treatment. The type of treatment your dermatologist tries will depend upon the age, size, and location of the keloids. Older and larger keloids are much more difficult to treat.

Treatment methods include injecting a cortisone-like substance directly into the keloid or removing the keloid surgically and following it up with the same cortisone injections. Surgical excision alone will make the keloid recur, possibly even larger than the original. Various types of sheeting applied for weeks or months, or freezing the area with liquid nitrogen or dry ice, may diminish the size and extent of the keloid. Good results for stubborn keloids have been reported using the carbon dioxide or pulsed dye laser.

Recap

- A keloid is an abnormal scar, a bizarre response to injury. Actually, it is an overgrowth of scar tissue.
- Keloids often develop over earlobes after ear-piercing, the upper arm following vaccinations, over appendectomy and gall bladder

operation scars, and on the chest area following acne bumps that have healed.

- If the keloid is small and inconspicuous, let it be. For larger lesions and those that are cosmetically unacceptable, your dermatologist can offer a variety of treatments.

STRETCH MARKS

Stretch marks are very thin scars that develop when the skin is stretched for a long period of time. This stretching strains the elastic fibers in the deeper layers of the skin to the point where they cannot regain their original resiliency. In simple terms, the skin doesn't "snap back" to its original shape.

The most common sites for stretch marks are the abdomen, hips, buttocks, thighs, and breasts. They usually show up at puberty (when young girls and boys fill out very rapidly), and with obesity and pregnancy. People who do repeated and strenuous exercises, like weight lifters and ballet dancers, often develop stretch marks. Less common factors include certain glandular disturbances; severe illnesses, such as scarlet fever and typhoid; and the use of salves and lotions containing strong cortisone-like preparations, when used in body folds over long periods of time.

Stretch marks are initially reddish or purple. After many months the color usually fades out and these shallow scars become white. There are *no* measures in the form of lotions, creams, or ointments that can decrease or erase these scars—so don't believe advertising claims that promise to get rid of them. Plastic surgeons may recommend a rather complicated surgical procedure, which involves cutting away a great deal of skin, tightening up the underlying muscles, and following all this up with dermabrasion. Before you contemplate such a drastic measure, keep in mind that the only problem they create is a cosmetic one.

You can take fairly simple measures to prevent stretch marks— maintain a stable weight and avoiding extreme tension on the skin.

Recap

- Stretch marks are very thin scars that commonly develop when the skin is stretched for a long period of time.

- People who do repeated and strenuous exercises, like weight lifters and ballet dancers, often develop stretch marks.
- There are *no* measures in the form of lotions, creams, or ointments that can decrease or erase these scars—so don't believe those ads that promise to get rid of them.

CELLULITE

A few years ago, a bestseller on the subject referred to cellulite (pronounced cell'-you-leet) as a "household word in Europe." It describes the "lumps, bumps, and bulges" that do not disappear with simple diet and exercise. What the book doesn't say is that cellulite affects practically every female of every age.

Cellulite is an invented disease. It is a "normal abnormality" that has tortured European women for many decades. The word cellulite was coined in the 1970s in European salons to describe the waffled-looking fat on women's buttocks and upper thighs. The proponents of this non-disease, seeking new markets for their advertising and useless remedies, have flooded the American market with "miracle" products and fraudulent claims.

To find out what cellulite looks like, make this pinch test: with your palms about four inches apart, press and squeeze together the outer part of your upper thigh. If the skin ripples and looks like a mattress, it means you have cellulite. It also probably means that you are a woman!

In a scientific investigation of almost a thousand women, cellulite occurred in practically all of them. It is not found in men who have the normal amount of male hormones (androgens). It is, however, found in men who have an androgen deficiency due to hormonal disease.

Cellulite is most common on the buttocks and thighs but can also occur on the lower part of the abdomen, the upper portions of the arms, and elsewhere. Contrary to reports in non-clinical literature, cellulite is not painful, nor is it the result of illness, miniskirts, or birth control pills.

What do hormones have to do with cellulite, and why do only

women have it? The following is a simplified, non-technical explanation:

The reason women have cellulite is that their skin is much thinner than that of men. As women get older, this thin skin becomes even thinner and looser, and clusters of fat cells begin to replace this lost skin. These fatty clusters high up in the skin are responsible for the mattress-like texture and the feel of cellulite.

What can you do about cellulite? Fad diet bestsellers, advertisements, and commercials would have you believe that diet, proper bowel function, breathing exercises, relaxation, yoga, massage, enzyme injections, liposuction, low power laser beams, iontophoresis, "mesotherapy," or the heralded "rice treatment" can eliminate this mark of womanhood. Don't believe them. Imagine pounding or massaging a glob of chicken fat. As hard or long as you knead, nothing is going to transform it!

The best way to prevent excessive so-called cellulite is to avoid becoming overweight. If you are overweight, slow and progressive weight loss and exercising to improve muscle tone in the buttocks and thighs may help reduce it. Female athletes, by the way, exhibit little or no cellulite.

Three factors counter cellulite, only one is within your control:

- choose a different set of grandparents.
- don't be a female.
- stay physically fit throughout your life.

It seems a pity that a form once considered "ideal" by such famous artists as Botticelli, Rubens, and Goya is no longer appreciated as chic or desirable.

Recap

- Cellulite is an invented disease. It is a "normal abnormality."
- Cellulite—really a fancy name for simple fat—is a sex-typical feature of women's skin and *not* a sign of disease.
- The best way to prevent excessive so-called cellulite is to avoid becoming overweight.

15
Problems of the Aging Skin

"A good leg will fall, a straight back will stoop, a black beard will turn white, a curl'd pate will grow bald, a fair face will wither...."
—Shakespeare: *Henry V*, Act V, scene ii, 168

An increasing proportion of our population is living longer, and as we've matured the consequences of time have become more apparent. The skin, hair and nails undergo characteristic changes with advancing age, dermatologic complaints increase steadily, and most people in their fifties and sixties have chronic skin problems.

There are two types of aging skin. One is a result of aging; the changes that occur in sun-protected skin. The other is a manifestation of chronic, sun-exposed skin, called photoaging. One we can do little about "the ineluctable modality of the visible"—the other we can prevent.

People of color—black and brown peoples—have stronger skins as a result of the protective melanin content of their pigment cells. If an African-American person has never been chronically exposed to the sun, and has never smoked, he or she will never exhibit a wrinkle, even until the age of eighty! Meanwhile, fair-haired, fair-skinned, blue-eyed Celtic women will wrinkle in their forties, even with only moderate exposures to the sun.

The integument of the darker-skinned individual will age much more slowly than his or her Caucasian neighbor. The skin of darker, southern Mediterranean and Arab people will age slower than the Scandinavian and fair-skinned northern European peoples.

People's appearance can alter their outlook, influence their self-perception, and affect their interpersonal relationships, particularly those enduring the changes of old age. We have been unable to slow these changes as yet. A significant degree of skin aging, however, is the end result of cumulative damage due to sun exposure.

Recent experiments have shown that it might be possible to reverse some degenerative processes. Experimental studies have indicated that the application of topical retinoic acid could eliminate some fine lines and wrinkles that have been caused by overexposure to the sun.

Dermatologists and plastic surgeons have been using injectable collagen implants—a simple, in-office procedure whereby the physician injects a modified bovine collagen into the upper layers of the dermis—to reduce cosmetically-unacceptable facial lines. Especially amenable to this type of therapy are the wrinkles of the forehead, the folds at the sides of the nose, and the area between the eyebrows. Unfortunately, the effect of this procedure is not permanent and injections must be repeated anywhere from six months to two years. Nonetheless, it offers a satisfactory spot treatment to those unwilling or unable to undergo more aggressive surgical operations. Some of the latest treatment remedies include a variety of laser procedures.

Aging skin undergoes changes in structure and function that significantly modify its appearance, and while these problems are medically insignificant and are nonthreatening, they are of profound cosmetic concern and detract from the quality of life for many older people.

Loss of elasticity, reduction in fat and moisture, changes in the supporting bone structure and muscles, wrinkles and increased dryness of the skin, changes in coloration, loss of scalp hair and growth of facial hair, and the emergence of skin growths are but a few of the many inevitabilities of advancing years.

Structural Changes in the Aging Skin

The normal, "young" epidermis—upper layer of the skin—furnishes a hardy, flexible barrier that prevents excessive water loss and protects us from an assortment of environmental insults.

In aging skin, certain changes occur. Some of these are:

- Overall thinning of the epidermis due to reduced hormone levels. This thinning is especially noted in the areas of sun exposure and results in the thin, shiny appearance of aged skin.
- A dwindling of moisture content of the skin and a reduction in the oiliness of the skin surface. This leads to dryness and roughness.
- A reduction in the protective barrier properties of the skin resulting in easily-induced irritant reactions.
- A decrease in the number of pigment cells in both exposed and non-exposed areas. This results in irregular, mottled pigmentation and the inability to tan as deeply or evenly as in earlier years.
- Changes in the function of these pigment cells in sunexposed areas induce "age spots" and patches of brown pigmentation on the neck of older women.
- In addition, there will be an increase of benign and malignant skin tumors: seborrheic keratoses, actinic keratoses, skin cancers, and other lesions, as mentioned in earlier chapters.

The function of the dermis—the lower layer of the skin—is to provide a tough matrix to support the many structures, which include blood vessels, nerves, and appendages that are embedded in it. Comprised chiefly of collagen and elastic fibers—the components that give the skin its texture and suppleness—the dermis decreases in thickness and density after the age of twenty, more so in females.

In the aging dermis, the total amount of collagen decreases steadily throughout adult life. In addition, the collagen becomes frayed at the edges and there is alteration and thickening of the collagen fibers. Aggravated by sun exposure, these changes result in the following:

- Skin deterioration. The skin becomes more mobile, and is easily picked up and pinched into folds. This is commonly observed over the tops of the hands. The skin becomes fragile and is easily torn. Wound healing is slowed.
- Permanent widening and tortuosity of the superficial capillaries which are seen conspicuously over the nose and cheeks.

239

- Black and blue marks. Loss of collagen support to the blood vessels make them susceptible to rupture from even the slightest trauma. Large discolored areas result from minor knocks, particularly over the tops of the hands and forearms where the skin has already been damaged by sun exposure.

Also as the skin ages the elastin network ages. The elastic fibers thicken and degenerate, resulting in:

- Wrinkles. The loss of elastic fibers, coupled with changes in the collagen, leads to fine wrinkles initially observed over the outer part of the eyes ("crow's feet"), forehead, and other sun exposed areas. Additional factors that contribute to wrinkles include the person's facial expressions ("the woman who doesn't smile never gets wrinkles"), the position in which the person sleeps, and whether the individual is a smoker. (Please see chapter on wrinkles.)
- Furrows develop at the site of facial expression lines. These are noted primarily over the upper lip in women and are also seen on the forehead, and the folds at the sides of the nose.
- Sagging and folds are commonly seen over the eyelids, neck, jaw, and arms.
- "Chicken neck." The skin of the sides of the neck has a ridged appearance with thickening around the openings of the hair follicles, making the skin look rippled. This phenomenon also appears over the temples and cheeks and is more common in women.
- "Peasant's neck." This yellowish, thick, weather-beaten, leathery skin of the back of the neck, with deep, crisscrossing furrows, is noted in men chronically exposed to the sun.

In addition, there is a decrease in the surface temperature, producing skin that is pale in appearance. The small blood vessels around the appendages—sweat glands, oil glands, and hair follicles—also diminish in density, resulting in decreased sweating, decreased oiliness, and thinning of the hair.

Care For the Aging Skin

What can we do to lessen the effects of the aging skin? Can we turn back the proverbial epidermal clock? Here are a few things to consider:

- Protect your largest organ from the ravaging rays of the sun.
- Keep your skin soft, smooth, and supple by massaging it (or, better yet, having it massaged) with emollient moisturizers. (Hairless mice treated with petrolatum have skin that is far superior to litter mates that have not been treated.) Your skin will become more resistant to physical and chemical insults if you keep it lubricated.
- A well-balanced diet and adequate fluid intake are necessary ingredients for a healthy older skin. Avoid excess alcohol consumption.
- Get enough sleep.
- If possible, avoid stress and tension.
- Don't smoke.
- Exercise! Inaction and sloth are enemies of healthy skin. As a result of the loss of collagen and elastic fibers, the body at constant rest will suffer dry, brittle, scaly and thin skin. Keep that circulation moving.

PHOTOAGING

A few notes on photoaging:

Photoaging is the combined effect of chronological aging and long-term sun damage on exposed parts of the body. In fair-skinned people with extensive sun exposure, photoaging may begin as early as the thirties and become more pronounced in the forties and fifties.

Features of photoaging include any or all of the following:

- Wrinkling.
- Roughness.
- Lax and leathery-looking.
- Irregular, spotty pigmentation.
- A sallow skin tone.
- Dilated capillaries (telangiectases).
- Clogged pores (blackheads and whiteheads).
- Actinic keratoses (rough, red precancerous growths).
- Easy bruising, particularly over the forearms and lower legs.

Retin-A and newer retinoids and alpha-hydroxy acids work on some people to lessen these wrinkles. Kinerase, in a cream and lotion, is an over-the-counter product that many women patients seem to like.

For more information on procedures used to reduce or eradicate the signs of aging skin, consult your dermatologist.

To prevent many of the signs of aging, stay out of the sun!

For further information about aging skin, log on to:
www.aad.org
1-888-462-DERM x22

Recap

- There are two types of aging skin: one is a result of chronological, intrinsic aging—changes that occur in sun-protected skin; the other is a manifestation of chronic, sun exposed skin—photoaging.
- The integument of the darker-skinned individual will age much more slowly than a Caucasian's.
- Aging skin undergoes alterations in structure and function that significantly modify its appearance. While these problems are often medically insignificant and are not life threatening, they are of profound cosmetic concern and detract from the quality of life for many older people.

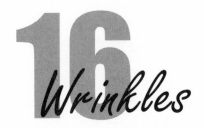

Wrinkles

Wrinkles—those bitter reminders of the aging process—are a natural phenomenon that occurs in all of us.

As we get on in years, the skin, for a number of reasons, begins to lose its elasticity, its flexibility, and its resiliency. It becomes thinner, fine lines develop, and then—horror of horrors—wrinkles.

What really happens to our skin, as we grow older? The sweat glands and oil glands, which for many years provided moisture and lubrication to the skin, get weary, work less, and diminish in size and number. The greater portion of the oils that have made the skin supple, as well as the sweat glands that have kept the cells plumped up and rounded, have for the most part disappeared, leaving the surface dry and cracked.

The fibers that support the skin begin to lose their strength and elasticity. Remember the old elevated trains? Just imagine that the pillars—the structures supporting the tracks—suddenly begin to bend, break, or crumble. What happens to the train and tracks? All fall down…That's basically what happens to the skin. The supporting collagen and elastic fibers deteriorate, and the skin begins to sag over the weakened and broken understructure.

There is also a reduction in the supply of beneficial hormones delivered to the skin cells. As a result, the fat pads in the skin begin to shrink, and certain fibers, which attach the skin to the muscles, relax and become weak, causing sagging and wrinkles.

Another type of aging skin is photoaging—a type of skin change due almost exclusively to sun exposure. Photoaged skin is wrinkled, yellowish, rough, lax, and leathery, with spotty pigmentation and fine veins over the cheeks and nose. "Normal" aged skin is thinner due to the aging process. There is loss of elasticity and a deepening of the normal expression lines.

At what age and how extensively one wrinkles is influenced by other factors as well:

- Heredity plays a major role in the production of wrinkles. People with thin skin—the Irish and Scottish, for example—age more rapidly than "thick-skinned" individuals. Black people rarely, if ever, develop wrinkles unless they have been exposed to the sun for a lifetime.

- Exaggerated facial expressions such as excessive laughing and frowning, and rough massages and facial exercises also weaken the elastic fibers and lead to premature wrinkling. The result will be horizontal lines of the forehead, "crow's feet" about the eyes, "laugh lines," and others. There is an old saying that contends, "the woman who never smiles, smokes or suns never develops wrinkles!"

- Sudden weight loss, due to diet or disease, also contributes to lines and wrinkles. After having been stretched out of shape for many years, the skin is unable to retract and so begins to hang in folds. This is comparable to what happens to a person's clothes after he or she loses a great deal of weight. They become loose, baggy, and begin to rumple. As our bones, fat and muscles shrink, the skin around them becomes loose.

- Excessive smoking appears to be a contributing factor in the formation of wrinkles. Did you ever notice how smokers screw up their faces to prevent smoke from getting in their eyes? This, coupled with a decrease in the circulation of blood to the facial skin, results in premature lines and wrinkles, particularly in lines of the upper lip ("whistler's wrinkles") and around the mouth.

- Exposure to the elements—heat, cold, wind, and especially sunlight—hastens and aggravates the natural aging process. You'll note that the skin of the buttocks shows none of the degenerative and aging changes we observe on the skin that's most exposed to the sun: the face, neck, hands, and forearms. The damage is palpable; the covered portions of your body are young, your sun exposed parts are old...

- Excessive washing and scrubbing, especially with harsh soaps and very hot water, contribute to breakage of the elastic fibers and tend to dissolve the essential oils that help nourish the skin.

Aging and wrinkling vary from person to person, so there is no hard and fast rule to pinpoint the exact decade when a person will begin to experience these hallmarks of decline. As a rule, however, in the forties and fifties, there is a progressive shrinking of body substance—bone, fat, muscle, and fluid—but *not* of the skin. This loss of tissue volume, coupled with the weakening of the elasticity of the skin, leads to sagging.

Sagging occurs first where the skin is thinnest: eyelids, neck, and jaw lines. Jowls develop, the neck becomes creased, lines begin to radiate from the mouth, and "crow's feet" and "bags" develop about the eyes. All this is a result of too much facial skin to cover the diminished amount of underlying tissue.

Can we do anything about wrinkles? Yes, but there are no types of cosmetic creams, potions, facial masks, exercises, acupuncture, laser treatments, injections of fetal cells, wrinkle ironing, or massages that can flatten out or permanently erase lines and wrinkles.

Mink oil, turtle oil, placenta extract and other expensive rejuvenating creams, "wrinkle creams," and facial masks offer nothing more than temporary relief from dryness, by lubricating and softening weather-beaten skin. Likewise, those facial saunas and the "electric needle" treatments have no lasting effect on dryness, lines, or wrinkles.

Masks, saunas, and the like can provide some psychological benefits, but let's not fool ourselves. Their permanent effect on the skin is zero. They cannot prevent, postpone or minimize the effects of the aging process. However, they probably won't harm you either—so if they make you feel good, enjoy them!

There are some things you can do to forestall the wrinkling process:

- Avoid the sun! I cannot stress this enough. In otherwise healthy people, sun exposure is the principal cause not only of wrinkles, aging skin, and other degenerative changes, but also skin cancers.

- Avoid extremes of heat and cold, and protect your face against the wind and rain and snow.
- Wash your face with a gentle soap or cleanser and avoid excessively hot water and harsh cleansers.
- Do not allow your weight to yo-yo. The constant expansion and contraction of the skin will only tire out the elastic fibers.
- No facial exercises or isometrics. When overdone, they can break down elastic fibers and the collagen in the skin.
- Cut down on smoking.

There are scores of products and procedures, old and new, that claim to remove or diminish the wrinkling and anti-aging processes. Divided into techniques, here are some examples:

Topical (surface) products:
- Vitamin C Cream (Cell-C)
- Active C (Laboratories La Roche Posay, France)
- NeoStrata SkinCeuticals line
- Alpha-hydroxy acids
- Beta-hydroxy acids
- Renova
- Retin-A Creams & Gels & Solutions
- Retin-A Micro
- Retinol in various products
- Avita Cream & Gel
- Kinerase (Cream and Lotion)
- Ubiquinone (Coenzyme-Q10)
  ...and dozens more

Injectable products
- Collagen (Zyderm and Zyplast)
- Silicone
- Botox (Botulinum toxin)
- Dermalogen (collagen protein taken from cadavers and injected)

Surgical procedures
- Dermabrasion
- Microdermabrasion—the outer layer of skin is stripped off with

a sandblasting technique of sodium bicarbonate crystals or aluminum hydroxide blown onto the skin and then vacuumed away. The old skin is purportedly replaced by smoother, younger skin.

- Chemical Peels. Removal of the upper layers of the skin with a chemical, usually trichloroacetic acid (TCA), salicylic acid, glycolic acid, resorcinol or phenol.
- Fat Transfer (Microliposuction). Your own fat is removed from your thigh, buttocks, or abdomen and injected into wrinkles at the sides of the nose and chin.
- Resurfacing Laser Surgery. High-energy lasers generate heat to remove the outer skin and wrinkles, reduce discoloration and improve leathery texture due to sun baked skin. This procedure is usually done around the eyes, the forehead and the upper lip. Types of lasers used are: Carbon Dioxide (CO_2); Erbium YAG; Nlite; CoolTouch™, Gore-Tex™. An inert substance that helps fill in lines in the lower third of the face

Check with your dermatologist about all the above. Try out some samples either from the dermatologist's office or the cosmetic counters. There is no "one good product" for everyone's face. Remember, you are unique. A product that your friend or sister might be using may cause you to burn, itch, or swell. If the product does agree with you, please be patient. Many work only after having used them for several weeks or months.

If you already have wrinkles, and if they are causing you great anguish, your only other options are cosmetic surgery or one of the above procedures. If you can afford it …the rewards can be great, but only you can decide whether you want to alter nature or let it take its course and grow old gracefully.…

For further information about wrinkles, log on to: www.aad.org
1-888-462-DERM x22
1-800-441-2737

Recap

- Aging skin undergoes alterations in structure and function that significantly modify its appearance. While these problems are often medically insignificant and non-life threatening, they are of profound cosmetic concern and detract from the quality of life for many older people.

- Heredity plays a major role in the production of wrinkles. People with thin skin—the Irish and Scottish, for example—age more rapidly than "thick-skinned" individuals. Black people rarely, if ever, develop wrinkles unless they have been exposed to the sun for a lifetime.

- Aging and wrinkling vary from person to person, so there is no hard and fast rule to pinpoint the exact decade when a person will begin to experience these hallmarks of decline.

17 Promising Home Remedies for Skin Disorders

The following home remedies—products usually found in your own kitchen—can help relieve the itching, pain, and discomfort of many skin ailments. Please be aware that not all work for everybody, and that if you have a stubborn, very itchy, or painful disorder for days or weeks, you should see your general physician or your dermatologist.

Yogurt—can be used for severe *itching* of the vulva due to *yeast infections* or to painful *cold sore* infections. Put 2 tablespoonfuls of unflavored yogurt on a handkerchief or sanitary napkin and apply it to the itchy or painful area. Leave on for several hours. Reapply as needed. Also excellent for *rectal itch*.

Eating yogurt—4 tablespoonfuls daily—can often prevent recurrent *canker sores*.

Tea Bags—excellent for *smelly and sweaty feet*. Take 2 tea bags and put them in a pint of boiling water for 15 minutes. Then remove the tea bags and pour the pint of strong, hot tea in a basin filled with 2 quarts of cool water. Soak your feet for 20 to 30 minutes daily for a week or ten days. No smell! No sweat! Repeat as often as needed.

Tea bags are also good for painful *canker sores* in the mouth. Immerse a tea bag in half a glass of tepid water until sopping wet. Remove the tea bag, squeeze out almost all the water, and then apply the tea bag directly to the canker sore. Hold it there for a few minutes. You may be pleasantly surprised.

Lemons (fresh)—good for removing *freckles* and *age spots*. Often as effective as expensive "fade creams." Cut a fresh lemon and squeeze the juice out of half in a small bowl. Using a cotton ball, wipe the affected spots with the lemon juice twice daily. Try this for 6 to 8 weeks. Repeat as necessary.

Onions—also can be used for removing *freckles* and *age spots*. Slice a red onion in half and rub on the spot twice daily. Continue until the spot or spots fade.

Onions are also good to prevent *insect bites* and *stings*. Eat a couple of raw onions (great with hamburgers!) daily during the summer. The insects will usually avoid you!

Garlic—along with the onions, eating garlic can prevent *mosquitoes* from attacking you.

Egg white—for those of you with facial *wrinkles* or large *pores*, the best and least expensive way of getting rid of them for about 2 hours (just before the party) is as follows:

About an hour before your party, wash your face thoroughly with a mild soap or cleanser. Let dry. Then beat up two egg whites into a meringue (until they are stiff). Apply the egg whites over your face and leave on for 20 to 30 minutes. Then rinse off with cool water (not hot, else you'll have scrambled eggs on your face!) and pat dry. Then put on your makeup. You'll be wrinkle free for about two hours. This is much less expensive than the 100-dollar-an-ounce anti-wrinkle creams, which also work for about 2 hours.

Meat tenderizer—excellent for *insect bites* and *stings*. For a mild bee or wasp sting, or for annoying mosquito and fleabites, make a paste of one-half teaspoon of unseasoned meat tenderizer with a few drops of water and apply directly to the bite or sting. You should obtain relief in a matter of minutes. For you outdoors people: always carry a bottle of the meat tenderizer with you when you plan a trip.

Ice cubes—an ice cube applied to a fresh *cold sore* will often abort the spread of the condition. Ice cubes are also good for *insect bites* and *stings*.

Duct tape—excellent for *warts* around and under fingernails. Apply 2 layers of the tape—one longwise and one around the finger up to the first joint—to make it airtight. Leave on for a week. Remove for 12 hours and reapply for another week. Keep doing this until the wart gets "tired" and disappears, leaving no mark or scar! (see page 31)

Nail polish—excellent for *chigger* bites. Apply the polish right on the bite and the chigger will suffocate and die.

Also, if you are allergic to nickel—earrings, jean snaps—and you don't want to purchase new items, you can coat the metals with clear nail polish. This will prevent the allergen from getting onto your skin. Since sweating may remove some of the lacquer from the metal after a time, reapply when necessary.

Glossary

Acne—a common skin eruption that usually appears on the face, chest, and back. In most cases, begins in adolescence when the oil glands enlarge and become inflamed. Characterized by blackheads, pimples, pustules, and occasionally cysts and scars.

Actinic—an adjective meaning "relating or pertaining to rays or beams of light."

Allergy—a hypersensitivity to a chemical, food, drug, metal, sunlight, or other substance.

Alopecia—hair loss.

Alopecia Areata—hair loss occurring in patches.

Alopecia Totalis—total hair loss of the scalp.

Alopecia Universalis—total hair loss of the entire body.

Anal Itch—proper term for Rectal Itch.

Androgen—a hormone that promotes male characteristics.

Antibiotic—a substance, such as penicillin and tetracycline that halts the growth of certain germs.

Antihistamine—a chemical used to alleviate itching in allergic reactions.

Aphthous Stomatitis—canker sores.

Ashy Skin—grayish looking skin in black people, which is nothing more than dry skin. It is *not* a sign of disease.

Athlete's Foot—a superficial fungous infection of the feet. Also known as ringworm of the feet.

Atopic Dermatitis—see Eczema.

253

Autoimmune Disease—a disease resulting from a disordered immune reaction in which antibodies are produced against one's own tissues, for example, lupus erythematosus.

Bacteria—germs capable of producing disease.

Benign—not malignant (noncancerous).

Birthmark—made up of blood vessels that collect in certain parts of the skin and occur at or shortly after birth. Also known as vascular birthmark.

Blackhead—a black-tipped plug of dried oil that has blocked a pore of an oil gland. The scientific name for this is comedone.

Blister—a swelling of the upper layers of the skin filled with fluid.

Boil—a painful and tender swelling of the skin caused by various bacteria. Also called a Furuncle.

Candidiasis—a common infection of the skin, mucous membranes, and nails caused by a yeast-like fungus called Candida. Also known as moniliasis.

Canker Sores—painful ulcers of the mouth or tongue. Also known as aphthous stomatitis.

Cellulite—a "normal abnormality" of almost all women characterized by the waffled-looking fat of the buttocks and upper thighs. It is a fancy name for plain fat. It is *not* a disease.

Chloasma—patchy excess pigmentation. See Melasma.

Cold Sore—a small blister on the face or other portion of the body caused by a Herpes virus. See Herpes.

Collagen—the generic name for a family of proteins that make up the major fibrous components of skin, tendons, ligaments, cartilage, and bone. It is what gives the skin its resilient and elastic quality.

Contact Dermatitis—an allergy or irritation on the skin resulting from exposure to certain substances (chemicals, plants, cosmetics, etc.).

Crabs—pubic **lice.**

Cradle Cap—seborrheic dermatitis of the scalp in infancy.

Crust—a scab or dried secretion on the surface of the skin.

Cuticle—the skin that is attached to the base of the nails.

Cyst—a skin tumor, almost always benign, filled with fluid or solid matter.

Dandruff—visible scaling of the scalp.

Depigmentation—loss of color or pigment.

Depilatory—a substance that removes hair.

Dermatitis—inflammation of the skin; an eczema.

Dermatosis Papulosa Nigra—tiny, smooth, raised, mole-like spots that appear on the face and neck of black people, usually inherited and darker than the surrounding skin. They never become malignant.

Diaper Rash—any eruption on an infant's buttocks, genital and anal areas, lower abdomen, and upper thighs that appears during the diaper-wearing stage.

Dimple Wart—a benign (friendly) tumor of the upper layers of the skin that is somewhat contagious. Also known as Molluscum Contagiosum.

Drug Eruption—a variety of rashes resembling measles; blisters; dry mouth; hair loss; and other manifestations on the skin, hair, nails and mucous membranes that develop as a result of the ingestion or injection of various types of medications.

Dry skin—a loose, unscientific term used to describe the scaly, flaky skin that is dry to the touch and less elastic than normal skin.

Eczema—synonym for dermatitis. Used by the dermatologist, it means atopic dermatitis.

Electrolysis—destruction of the hair root with an electric current.

Endocrine Glands—certain hormone-producing glands (thyroid, adrenal, etc.).

Epidermis—the outer layer of the skin.

Fever Blister—synonym for cold sores or herpes.

Follicle—a tiny, sac-like structure out of which the hair grows.

Folliculitis—a hair follicle infection.

Freckles—small spots of pigmentation over the face and shoulders in some people (often redheads) which get darker when exposed to the sun.

Frostbite—the sharp, painful sensations that result from severe cold injury.

Fungus—a microorganism (actually a miniature plant) that is responsible for various fungous infections (athlete's foot, jock itch, tinea versicolor, and others).

Furuncle—see Boil.

Genital herpes—cold sores of the genital region.

Hemangioma—a common vascular birthmark that appears at or shortly after birth.

Herpes Simplex—cold sores. An inflammation of the skin caused by a virus and characterized by small, itchy blisters on a red base. Also known as fever blisters.

Herpes Zoster—shingles.

Hirsutism—excessive growth of hair in the areas of the skin, such as the face and chest, that are usually reserved for male hair growth.

Hives—an allergic reaction characterized by itching and burning wheals (welts) on the skin.

Hyperpigmentation—excessive coloration of the skin.

Hypersensitivity—the tendency to be allergic.

Hypertrichosis—a disorder where unwanted hair is more or less generalized in distribution.

Hypopigmentation—decreased coloration of the skin.

Ichthyosis—a dry, rough, scaly, hereditary skin disorder. Also called "fishskin disease."

Infestation—the invasion of the skin by a mite or parasite. Scabies and lice are infestations.

Impetigo—an infectious disease of the skin caused by the streptococcus or staphylococcus germs and characterized by "stuck-on," honey-colored crusts.

Integument—the skin.

Involute—having the margins rolled inward.

Itch—an irritation of the skin that causes a desire to scratch.

Jock Itch—an itching and inflammation of the groins, usually caused by a fungus. Also known as ringworm of the groin.

Keloid—an enlarged or overgrown scar.

Keratosis—a scaly, crusted, wart-like growth.

Keratosis Pilaris—a common rash over the backs of the arms and thighs that looks and feels like a cheese grater. It is a harmless condition and usually improves in the warmer weather. It appears to be a marker for those who have eczema.

Laser—an abbreviation of Light Amplification by Stimulated Emission of Radiation. It is used in dermatological therapy for a variety of disorders, including warts, cancers, and cosmetic surgical procedures.

LE—an abbreviation for lupus erythematosus.

Lice—parasites that cause itching.

Lichenification—a thickening and darkening of the skin, with accentuated skin markings, as a result of constant scratching.

Lichen Planus—an itchy skin rash characterized by flat, violet-colored bumps that generally appear on the wrists, ankles, and lower back.

Lupus Erythematosus—a collagen disease that can involve any organ of the body. When it involves the skin, it appears as disc-shaped, red, scarred patches on the face and scalp. Same as LE.

Malignant—cancerous.

Melanin—the brownish-black pigment produced in the skin.

Melanocyte—a cell that produces melanin.

Melanoma—a dangerous malignant tumor of the skin that spreads rapidly and is often fatal.

Melasma—a brownish, mottled pigmentation of the skin, usually seen on the face of women. Also known as chloasma.

Miliaria—prickly heat.

Mite—a parasite of the skin. Scabies is caused by a mite.

Mole—a birthmark—or nevus; a pigmented growth on the skin, with or without hair.

Molluscum Contagiosum—see dimple wart.

Monilia—a yeast-like fungus responsible for many rashes, especially in the groins. See Candida.

Nails—specialized horny extensions of the skin made up of keratin.

Nevus—a mole.

Nevus Flammeus—port-wine stain.

Nit—the egg of a louse.

Oral—by mouth.

Paronychia—an inflammation of the soft tissue around the nails.

Pediculosis—louse infestation.

Perleche—cracks in the corners of the mouth.

Photosensitivity—an exaggerated sensitivity to light.

Pityriasis Alba—occurring primarily in childhood—usually from ages 8 to 12—it consists of light patches over the cheeks and, occasionally, other areas such as the arms and neck. It also appears to be a marker for those who have eczema.

Pityriasis Rosea—a common skin disorder that begins with a solitary patch of redness and scaling and evolves over a period of about two weeks in a fairly generalized rash. It is not contagious.

Plantar Wart—a wart on the bottom—sole—of the foot.

Poison Ivy—a three-leafed plant that is commonly responsible for poison ivy dermatitis.

Port-wine Stain—a flat, reddish-purple mark that appears most often on the face and on the back of the neck. A type of birthmark. Also called nevus flammeus.

Postherpetic Neuralgia—a severe, sometimes relentless pain that follows an attack of shingles. Occurs primarily in the older population groups.

Prickly Heat—a common disorder of the sweat apparatus that arises when the free flow of sweat to the surface of the skin is obstructed.

Pruritus—itching.

Pseudofolliculitis Barbae—see "Razor Bumps."

Psoriasis—a common chronic, inflammatory skin disease characterized by scaly patches.

Pustule—a pus-filled pimple.

Pyoderma—an impetigo-like infection of the skin accompanied by weeping, oozing, and painful crusts.

Rash—an eruption on the skin.

"Razor Bumps"—ingrown hairs of the beard in black men. The technical name for this is pseudofolliculitis barbae.

Rectal Itch—itching of the anal area. The correct term is anal itch.

Ringworm—a common term for a fungous infection of the skin and scalp. Athlete's foot is a ringworm infection of the feet.

Rosacea—a chronic skin disorder of middle-aged people, characterized by redness of the face accompanied by acne-like pimples and pustules.

Scabies—an intensely itchy, contagious skin condition caused by a mite.

Scar—a permanent mark left on the skin following a wound or surgical procedure.

Sebaceous Gland—a gland in the skin that produces sebum (oil).

Seborrheic Dermatitis—an inflammation of the sebaceous glands producing yellow, greasy scales primarily over the scalp and face.

Sebum—the oily material produced by the sebaceous glands.

Shingles—herpes zoster. A viral infection caused by a virus and characterized by itching, pain, and a rash on one side of the body.

Skin Tags—small, fleshy, benign growths that are often seen in the armpits and around the neck.

Stretch Marks—very thin scars that commonly develop when the skin is stretched for a long period of time.

Tinea Capitis—ringworm of the scalp.

Tinea Versicolor—a "friendly" fungous infection of the skin characterized by fawn-colored, scaly patches over the chest and back.

Topical—surface (as in topical medication as opposed to internal medication).

Tumor—a new growth. A tumor can be benign (friendly) or malignant (unfriendly). A wart is a benign tumor; a melanoma is a malignant tumor.

Ulcer—an open sore or wound.

Urticaria—hives.

Vitiligo—a skin disorder characterized by patchy loss of pigment.

Wart—a contagious growth on the skin or mucous membranes caused by a virus.

Wen—a smooth, round, dome-like soft or moderately hard tumor of the scalp filled with greasy, cheese-like, odoriferous material.

Wheal—a welt or hive.

Whitehead—a small plug that blocks the skin pore; actually, a closed blackhead.

Winter Itch—see dry skin.

"Zits"—common acne pimples.

Index